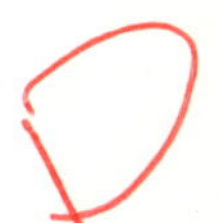

THE EIGHTEENTH-CENTURY CAMPAIGN TO AVOID DISEASE

By the same author

INTERNATIONAL GOVERNMENT FINANCE AND THE AMSTERDAM CAPITAL MARKET, 1740–1815

POPULATION THOUGHT IN THE AGE OF THE DEMOGRAPHIC REVOLUTION

THE EIGHTEENTH-CENTURY CAMPAIGN TO AVOID DISEASE

James C. Riley

Professor of History
Indiana University

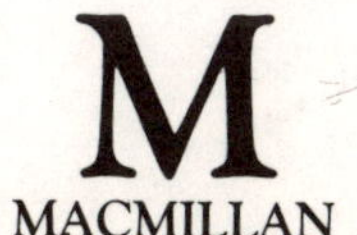

First published 1987

Published by
THE MACMILLAN PRESS LTD
Houndmills, Basingstoke, Hampshire RG21 2XS
and London
Companies and representatives
throughout the world

Printed in Hong Kong

British Library Cataloguing in Publication Data
Riley, James C.
The eighteenth-century campaign to avoid disease.
1. Epidemics—History—18th century 2. Public health—History—18th century
I. Title
614.4'09'033 RA649
ISBN 0-333-40622-2

For Anneke

Everyone knows that the milieu
is the first, the principal
and even the only cause of
epidemic diseases . . .

FOURNIER-CHOISY

Contents

Introduction

In the Hippocratic tradition the physician is urged to become familiar with the milieu of man and disease: 'Whoever wishes to pursue the science of medicine in a direct manner must first investigate the seasons of the year and what occurs in them'.[1] Reading further in *Airs, Waters and Places*, and in the first and third books of *Epidemics*, we discover that the student of medicine must also examine winds, waters, site, soil, diet, and other characteristics of a locale which influence its diseases. Doing these things, the travelling Greek physician would have less opportunity to be surprised by the endemic or epidemic diseases encountered from place to place. The physician is to observe these things, but Hippocratic tradition did not suggest that environmental circumstances influencing local diseases might themselves be modified. The diseases could be treated. But the environment was a datum, to be viewed fatalistically.[2] A passive attitude remained strong in the sixteenth and seventeenth centuries.[3]

This Hippocratic view of disease and its environment has always exercised a large influence over medicine in the West. What has waxed and waned is not so much attachment to it as the medical approach to the problem of endemic and epidemic (as distinct from individual) manifestations of disease. In the second half of the seventeenth century European physicians in several locations began to rethink the ways in which they were accustomed to understand large-group disease. Adhering still to classical insights, they shifted emphasis away from Galen and the attribution of disease to disorder within man toward a revived Hippocratic notion of disease as the product of disorder between man and the environment.[4] Revivals of this sort had occurred before. On this occasion, however, the revival coincided with certain fresh approaches to the study of man and the environment, and with a rapidly expanding body of information about these things. The fresh approaches and the new data evolved into a medical theory of endemic and epidemic (especially epidemic) disease. This step broadened and prolonged interest in the association between milieu and disease, and created an expectation. Convinced already that epidemics might be explained by the environmental conditions that preceded them, eighteenth-century physicians believed that they stood on the verge of discovering how the causal relation worked. Knowing the cause, they could intervene – not only to combat the effects of this association in the patient, but also to impede contact between man and disease-causing agents.

Around the middle of the eighteenth-century the Hippocratic tradition underwent a fundamental change, stepping away from the fatalism that had for so long characterised the physician's attitude toward the environmental causes of disease. No longer might individual patients merely be treated and perhaps cured. No longer would the quarantine be the principal technique of prevention. The epidemic itself could be avoided. This is the origin not of medicine (which is the treatment of ills), nor exclusively of preventive medicine (which is the attempt to foresee and forestall disease). It is the origin of a medicine of avoidance and prevention, a medicine that sought to show mankind which disease-conducive circumstances to evade, and to determine what aspects of the environment might be modified to weaken or eliminate their capacity to cause disease.

In that day physicians concerned with large-group manifestations of disease construed the new things they sought to do as an attack on mortality. By detaching man from disease-ridden and disease-conducive sites and situations, they would disrupt the epidemic cycle at that point at which man received or absorbed pathogenic influences from the environment. In retrospect we can recognise this as an attack against both mortality and morbidity. The medicine of avoidance would protect man from some often fatal diseases, but it sought also to elude epidemic disease in general, to avoid influenza and malaria as well as smallpox and typhus.

Looking about themselves, these physicians saw afresh the habitat of man. It was a habitat of stagnant waters and steaming marshes and fetid cesspits; of narrow, airless, and filth-ridden streets and passages; of hovels and grand buildings without ventilation; of the dead incompletely isolated from the living. It was, we can now see, a habitat in which the microorganisms of disease (and the living vectors that transmit those microorganisms and other pathogenic matter) thrived. We must pause for a moment to try to recapture these scenes, to recreate, or to create for the first time, in our mind's eye the images of refuse and waste strewn here and there that filled the eyes of the seventeenth-century European, that spring so vividly from the pages of Samuel Pepys' diary. Neither the city nor the small town nor the village escaped this, for few of them possessed or used the most elementary techniques for disposing of the waste of man and nature. Although we cannot now verify such a supposition, it is inescapable to suppose that fleas, lice, houseflies, mosquitoes, rodents, and other small animals and insects which act as living disease vectors and vector hosts existed in stupendous numbers in these conditions. It was the golden age of these organisms. The population of Europe had arrived at its highest historical density – some 110 million around 1700 and some 140 million around 1750[5] – before any widespread adoption of measures designed to dispose of the refuse of existence or to control pests. The human population had thus reached a peak in its capacity to generate conditions in which such organisms thrive, and in the density of human settlement in contact with refuse in the cities, the numerous small towns, and the villages of Europe.

The physician let his gaze fall more often and more carefully upon man's milieu. In this eighteenth-century form of disease control, the physician would put the environment under surveillance in order to detect its disease-conducive qualities, and to discover how to avoid them. He did not discern either microorganism or vector. The mechanism causing epidemic disease this physician saw as a complex of environmental conditions and forces, a particular aggregation of climatic and environmental circumstances. To counter the aggregation, to intrude upon its capacity to provide the occasion for epidemics, the physician of the environment would either remove man from such sites and complexes, cleanse the site, or otherwise disrupt the complex. The measures of principal utility seemed to be drainage, lavation, ventilation, and reinterment.

To pursue the eighteenth-century form of this idea – that epidemic diseases arise from the environment – is the goal of this book. The pursuit will take two directions. In the first, the issues lie in both the social history of medicine and the history of medical theory and thought. They deal with the hypothesis of a disease–environment association, with the specification of disease-causing environmental factors and forces and of efficacious reactions (drainage, lavation, ventilation, and reinterment), and with overt and covert lines of thought that made these ideas seem persuasive. Here also the spread of the idea of an environment–disease association in its particular late seventeenth- and early eighteenth-century form will be followed across Europe and into some parts of the non-European world inhabited by Europeans. Most of the evidence about these ideas and their implementation will deal with Britain, France, the Low Countries, and the Germanies. But evidence will also be drawn from areas on the periphery of this region – Sweden, Russia, Italy, Spain – and from North America, the West Indies, and the East Indies. The actions and the new optimism about the efficacy of medicine follow from the ideas. We shall notice quickly enough, however, that the concern of the physician of the environment concentrated on disease and environmental pathogens rather than upon the diseased. To be precise, this direction deals with the social history of *disease* and the history of disease theory.

It is this gaze toward the milieu that most closely links old regime medicine to the movement of ideas outside medicine. In assessing the role of the environment as a source of disease, in recording the signs and symptoms of the association, in rethinking the foundations for explaining disease, and in proposing to find an efficacious medicine, the physician's thought ran parallel to the thought of students of astronomy, botany, chemistry, political institutions, criminal law, economics and many other fields. In this realm medicine both drew from and contributed to the development of ideas, which is usually identified with the Enlightenment. But the *philosophes* of the Enlightenment were often scornful of medicine. Realising this, and discovering the strength of tradition in the medicine of the environment, we shall understand that not only the thinkers who regarded themselves as enlightened shed pessimism and passivity for optimism and action.

The second direction to be investigated is how this medicine of the environment influenced epidemic disease, and thus mortality and morbidity, in a century in which mortality rates are known to have diminished but from undetermined causes.[6] A mortality decline began in the seventeenth century, continued in the eighteenth and nineteenth century, and has not yet ended. To all appearances it began in western and central Europe, and first took the form of a decline in the incidence of virulent infectious diseases. Outside this region high mortality rates remained common for a longer period. The plan to attack the environmental sources of disease was also a cosmopolitan phenomenon, for evidence of it is to be found across Europe. It too emerged in western and central Europe, where there were more physicians, and where therefore there was more learned interest in epidemiology. Before the late nineteenth- and early twentieth-century epidemiological transition, from infectious to chronic degenerative diseases, the leading cause of high mortality rates coincides with the source of the eighteenth-century physician's concern – infectious disease in epidemic form.

The sources consulted for this book thus lead to a new explanation for part of the European mortality decline – that this medicine of avoidance and prevention actually diminished mortality and morbidity, if often for reasons and in ways that physicians themselves did not understand or intend. One of the objectives of this book is to show why this explanation should join other ideas about why there was a decline in the death rate: improvements in nutrition, climatic amelioration, specific medical advances (chiefly smallpox inoculation), a decreasing virulence of microorganisms, and changes in the biology of microorganisms. If these hypotheses could account for the mortality decline, new explanations would not be needed. But they do not, or – in the case of the biological hypotheses – they do so only in a manner which no way has yet been found to test.

The explanation advanced here suggests that mortality declined, and more specifically that the number and severity of epidemics fell, because epidemiological action – drainage, lavation, ventilation, reinterment, and other similar measures – reduced human contact with disease-causing pathogens in the environment. The leading means was the disruption of conditions in which vectors carrying pathogenic matter (such as the housefly that transmits typhoid and dysentery) and vectors playing a necessary role in the biological development and transmission of pathogens (such as the mosquito that hosts the malaria pathogen) thrived. Whereas eighteenth-century physicians believed they were attacking the direct and immediate causes of disease, I believe they were actually attacking disease indirectly and unwittingly, through the vectors that transmit it.

This hypothesis can be tested in at least two directions. Mortality can be compared in improved and unimproved sites to discover whether the improvements coincide with reductions in the death rate. Some tests of this nature have been conducted by historians, and some were conducted in the eighteenth century. These will be discussed here. They are inconclusive, not because they report conflicting results, but because the controls over site – and over factors other than the presence or absence of specific eighteenth-century style improvements – are imperfect. Moreover, such tests are not numerous. They support the hypothesis, and they point up the usefulness, where data can be found, of performing additional (and more thoroughly controlled) tests.

A second potential area of testing is to investigate whether in fact morbidity moved parallel to mortality, declining during the eighteenth century, and especially from the 1740s on, when environmental modifications were introduced in large numbers. If these modifications successfully diminished mortality in the way hypothesised here, they should also have reduced morbidity rates. We know very little about morbidity in this period, and what we do know emerges almost exclusively from mortality data. It is especially about non-fatal instances of sickness, epidemic and non-epidemic, that we are ignorant. We may suppose that the high mortality rates of the seventeenth and early eighteenth century – rates usually between 25 and 40 per 1 000 per annum – coincided with a high incidence of morbidity. We may suppose also that mortality was high in part because of the debilitating effects of diseases that are ordinarily not fatal, and that many people died while suffering from the combined effects of two or more diseases. If early modern European morbidity could be readily explored, we should expect to discover both the prevalence of disease, and the overlapping of diseases, 'infection with infection . . . a synergism between disease and disease'.[7] The vigour of the population, and the resistance of the population to other diseases, commonly fatal or not, may thus have been diminished by a morbidity complex, a situation in which epidemics and diseases in general overlapped one another, and in which secondary infections played a large part in immediate and deferred mortality. It is this line of testing that I wish to pursue in future research. And it is this line of inquiry to which the physician's concern with the environmental causes of disease calls attention. This is so because the environment was seen as a source of all manner of disease, and because in eighteenth-century medicine diseases continued to be seen as overlapping and merging forces rather than distinct entities.

The medicine of avoidance and prevention did not die at the end of the eighteenth century. But it did change character. What earlier had been an open-ended search for information about man's habitat combined with a campaign to take certain measures to modify the environment began to ossify. We know the medicine of the environment in the nineteenth century pejoratively, as the miasmic theory of disease. It was a theory that led to certain unambiguous advances in epidemiology – for example, John Snow's identification of an association between cholera and proximity to the great sewage stream that many European rivers had become. But it was also a theory whose followers resisted modification and innovation, specifically resisting reintroduction of the contagion theory of disease transmission directly from individual to individual, and introduction of the germ theory of disease. I have elected to suspend the story at the point of ossification, at the point at which subsequent contributions more often fortified existing presuppositions than added new knowledge or raised grounds for doubting environmentalist-cum-miasmic assumptions. The later story is well known.[8] It is the eighteenth-century form of epidemiology that deserves to be recognised and studied, and it is the problem of explaining the eighteenth-century regression of mortality that is most intriguing.

I wish to coin a term to stand for this eighteenth-century form of epidemiology. The term is 'environmentalism'. The scholarly literature has often touched on eighteenth-century epidemiology, and it suggests many phrases to describe the study of the link between environment and disease. Alfred Haviland chose the term 'iatro-meteorology', August Hirsch 'geographical and historical pathology', Kenneth Dewhurst 'environmental and social medicine'.[9] Folke Henschen has used the phrase 'historico-geographical pathology' to distinguish the history of diseases from the history of medicine or of physicians.[10] Michel Foucault coined a distinction between a 'medicine of climates and [a medicine of] places'.[11] Each phrase refers to things that overlap, but only in part. I prefer a variation on Dewhurst's term, one adopted also in 1979, by L. J. Jordanova – 'environmental medicine' (or, for the sake of simplicity, 'environmentalism').[12] In using this word and the phrase 'medicine of the environment' I do not wish to confuse eighteenth-century attitudes toward the environment with twentieth-century ecological or environmentalist thinking. After all, the idea of a pathogenic environment contrasts sharply with the late twentieth-century conception of a benign if not sympathetic environment sometimes made pathogenic by man's abuse of it. For me the word 'environmentalism' refers to nothing more than what W. F. Bynum has called 'environmental factors in the aetiology of disease'.[13] This is a subject of investigation that cuts across several modern realms of specialisation – epidemiology, biometeorology or medical climatology, and medical geography. Each field has a rich but inadequately remembered eighteenth-century background.

This is a history stressing continuity in a branch of the discipline, medical history, in which the literature focuses on discontinuities distinguishing eighteenth- from nineteenth-century medicine. Shryock, Ackerknecht, Vess, and Foucault, to mention only a few writers, have detected in the era of the French Revolution changes in practice so sweeping that they warrant the label 'revolutionary'.[14] This sense of radical discontinuity is appropriate, I think, for the medicine of the individual. But it is inappropriate for the medicine of aggregate man, which is the subject of this book. There the revolution came somewhat earlier, when pessimism and passivity gave way to optimism and action.

Many physicians wrote in the seventeenth and eighteenth century about the problems of large-group manifestations of disease. Their writings cannot all be mentioned, and need not all be mentioned. In selecting those authors I would discuss here, I have followed three techniques. First, I have been interested especially in those physicians who stepped back from the individual patient and looked at their patients (or at the diseased in general) as a group. Second, I have taken note of the frequent text and footnote references in the eighteenth-century medical literature in an effort to read the books and essays that the environmentalists themselves were reading. John Arbuthnot's *An Essay Concerning the Effects of Air on Human Bodies* illustrates this cataloguing of references and the cosmopolitan nature of discourse about the environmental causes of disease. Third, I have looked for those physicians who most effectively expressed an idea, and thus often I report on an idea not from the earliest mention that can be discovered, but from the writings of that physician who articulated it most clearly.

Several people have contributed to this book, and I wish to thank them for their assistance. The first person to read the manuscript, and to suggest that it might have some interest, was Erwin H. Ackerknecht. Other equally astute medical and public health historians also attempted to show me how the argument might be made more effective, and to point me toward sources that I had not encountered. For that I thank Ann Carmichael, Genevieve Miller, Abraham Lilienfeld, and Ann La Berge. Similar help from a different perspective was provided by Michael Flinn and Eric Jones. This book has been shaped very much by their suggestions, although I do not wish to hold them responsible for the way in which I decided in the end to arrange the narrative, or the judgements I reached.

This book also owes much to the generosity and cordial assistance of librarians, especially to Dorothy Hanks of the Historical Division of the National Library of Medicine, and to the patient staff of the Indiana University Interlibrary Loan Service.

JAMES C. RILEY

1 The Revival and Refinement of Hippocratic Ideas

Observations of this Kind, when regularly made for a long Series of Years, in one and the same Place, more certainly discover the Constitution of the Atmosphere in that Country, the reigning Disorders, their Successions, Relations one to another, and even the very Method of Cure.

Huxham

But tho' abstinence from Air is not, the Sort of Air which they use, is in the Power of a great many people: And as the Choice of Air is a Subject about which a Physician's Advice is often demanded, its Nature and different Qualities is a proper one of his studies.[1]

Arbuthnot

INTRODUCTION

Eighteenth-century physicians admired their seventeenth-century colleague Thomas Sydenham, 'the English Hippocrates', because Sydenham's work and reputation seemed so rich in inspiration. Sydenham had recommended the compilation of case histories, which contributed significantly to the eighteenth-century effort to classify diseases. Sydenham had urged the importance of clinical observation at a time when most physicians relied on a Galenic and humoural theory of disease and considered it more important to attain a proper theoretical understanding of illness and health than to draw inferences from clinical experience. Sydenham thus seemed to have anticipated another eighteenth-century interest, one often identified with the Dutch physician Boerhaave, in clinical observation. To Sydenham aetiology was less interesting than therapy. He turned away from the microscope, from dissection, and from counting and measuring, and focused instead on finding ways to identify effective remedies. To the eighteenth-century physician, under attack for the failure of therapy, Sydenham seemed to have foreseen the need for an efficacious medicine. And Sydenham seemed to his successors to have revived the Hippocratic idea that the seeds of disease lie both within and outside the body – that disease, especially when large numbers of people are affected, finds its origins in man's habitat. This reaffirmation of Hippocratic wisdom the eighteenth-century physician took to be the inspiration for a revised explanation of endemic and epidemic disease.

In fact, Sydenham had written a little about a great many things, so that it is difficult to find a developed argument about some of these issues. As an admirer of Hippocrates, he accepted environmental factors as causal agents behind disease. But he did not regard the study of such matters in detail as an issue of great importance, for he preferred to concentrate on therapy. Furthermore, Sydenham's lack of interest in counting and measuring conflicted with eighteenth-century interest in quantifying the signs and symptons of both man and man's environment.

The eighteenth-century environmentalist overlooked these contradictions and inconsistencies, finding a simple line of succession to his own interest in environmental causes of disease. Hippocrates was taken to have discovered the verity, and Sydenham to have revived interest in it. What is more, both Hippocrates and Sydenham were taken to have set forth the steps necessary to discover and specify the relationship between environment and disease. The eighteenth-century physician, secure in the strength of classical authority if inclined sometimes to prefer one authority (Hippocrates) to another (Galen), thus professed to rely less upon novelty than upon tradition.

In truth, this was partly a myth. Not only Sydenham but also Hippocrates had had remarkably little to say about the relationship between environment and disease, and had given remarkably little guidance in what precisely the environmentalist should do to understand disease, or treat it better. Many other sources inspired the medicine of the environment. Some of these lie among Sydenham's contemporaries and associates. The eighteenth-century references to Sydenham thus subsumed the work of several physicians and physicists who had formulated the details, and the terms, of environmentalist theory. Some sources derived from links to Hippocrates independent of Sydenham, links to be found in the Renaissance campaign for urban cleanliness and in the traveller's curiosity about the reigning diseases and environmental characteristics of territory new to Europeans.[2] Other sources lie within the mind of the eighteenth-century physician, or outside medicine altogether. The purpose of this chapter is to introduce these sources, especially the medical sources, and to explain the assumptions about disease to which they led. This chapter will also extract the main points the sources make about how the behaviour of the physician should be modified.

The Hippocratic Tradition

'Whoever wishes to pursue the science of medicine . . . must first investigate the seasons of the year and what occurs in them.' Observe and reflect upon winds, drinking waters, site, elevation, soil, climate, astrological features, and diet, the better to understand diseases and treatments.[3] To illustrate this advice, *Airs, Waters and Places* offered examples of four sites and their relevant environmental features. One, for instance, was 'sheltered from the east winds', but its drinking water was 'unclean and impure' because of 'the air that prevails at dawn'.[4]

Eighteenth-century physicians believed that Hippocrates had set forth a persuasive case that certain environmental complexes, certain 'constitutions', cause (or are conducive to) disease. But they found in Hippocrates no detailed evidence about how the association operates. Nor did they find in Hippocratic tradition a satisfactory explanation for the inconstancy of the disease–environment relationship – for example, the appearance of the same disease in different environmental complexes, or the failure of the same disease always to appear in what seemed to be the same environmental complex.

If Hippocratic tradition failed to provide a detailed theory of the environmental forces behind disease, it did nevertheless introduce a number of specific ideas about disease-causing and disease-conducive circumstances. For example, it associated standing water with diarrhoea, chronic quartan fever, dysentery, and other disorders; it held that 'the waters that flow from high places and from earthy [rather than rocky] hills are the best and healthiest'.[5] In addition to asserting that epidemics may be caused by climatic conditions, this part of the Hippocratic tradition held that cultural traits may also be causal agents of disease, and explained cultural traits for the most part by reference to climate and diet. As an eighteenth-century physician reported, 'Hippocrates observ'd, That the Inhabitants of moist Countries were bloated, leucophlegmatick, and dull'.[6] Wesley Smith has pointed out that there were several Hippocratic traditions. In another of them, Hippocrates appeared as the model observer of things.[7]

In the seventeenth century, these elements of a theory would be refined and strengthened. Whereas these parts of the Hippocratic tradition drew attention especially to endemic disease,[8] the seventeenth-century refinement would bring epidemic disease more forcefully into consideration. Whereas the features of site and climate described in the Hippocratic tradition (for the most part unalterable things) were described in order to show the travelling physician what to expect, the seventeenth-century refinement of these ideas would lead to a search for how to avoid or prevent endemic and epidemic disease. Throughout the attachment of the name of the great Greek physician to this search into the environment would lend credibility to the radical procedure of shifting the physician's gaze from the patient to the patient's habitat.

Seventeenth-Century Additions

In the 1670s the English physician and political economist William Petty explained how he proposed to undertake a general study of the resources of Britain, the Dutch Republic, and France: 'The Method I take to do this, is not yet very usual; for instead of using only comparative and superlative Words, and intellectual Arguments, I have taken the course (as a Specimen of the Political Arithmetick I have long aimed at) to express my self in Terms of *Number*, *Weight*, or *Measure*'.[9] Having counted some financial resources, for example, Petty would estimate the relative and potential strength of states. In other writing he exposed the technique of quantification as applied to demographic and medical matters. In 'Observations upon the Dublin-Bills of Mortality, 1681 and the State of that City', Petty offered a nosology under three headings (contagious, acute, and chronic) and twenty-four disease categories. Mortality records should be arranged according to cause, and then totalled within each parish according to these subdivisions 'in Order to know how the different Situation, Soil, and Way of living in each Parish, doth dispose Men to each of the said three [disease headings]'.[10]

Petty proposed to count diseases in order to detect the environmental complex behind them. Simultaneously other physicians and natural scientists proposed to observe and count the features of the habitat directly. As a scientific activity this is a familiar part of the story of scientific curiosity in the seventeenth century. Physicians, proto-environmentalists or not, shared this curiosity. In the eighteenth century they would practise what Petty had recommended, observing and counting diseases and environmental features, in order to search for associations between them. The mathematics of environmentalism thus assumes considerable importance. It was, it now seems, a simple mathematics. But the idea of systematic aggregations of disease data, and quantification of the characteristics of climate and habitat, was new. Furthermore, the sources are abundant in their testimony of mathematical inexpertise – the failure of even expert calculators to add correctly a column of numbers. In the first instance, therefore, the mathematics Petty proposed to bring to the service of the physician was elementary even if the learned populace was still imperfectly numerate, imperfectly adept at using numbers and performing the four basic arithmetic procedures of adding, subtracting, multiplying, and dividing. These were not new procedures, but they were unfamiliar to many people. Petty had learned much about them from his friend, the merchant John Graunt, and evidently contributed to Graunt's ideas about what should be counted, as expressed in Graunt's *Natural and Political Observations . . . made upon the Bills of Mortality* (1662).

In the second instance, however, the mathematics necessary to explore the question of the environment–disease association was new, and intricate. Petty would count historical phenomena. To use such tallies to make predictions, which Petty wished to do, required mathematical expectation. An aspect of probability theory worked out in the 1650s by Blaise Pascal and Christiaan Huygens,[11] among others, mathematical expectation showed how to combine the principle of a fair lottery (expressed as a simple algebraic formula) with historical experience to interpret fragmentary evidence about the present or to forecast future patterns. Using this formula, mortality records giving cause of death could be made to yield a quantitative prediction of the probability that any future death would be from the same cause. Similarly, the historic ratio of deaths per annum to the living population could furnish a prediction of the likely number of deaths in a current population, or the likelihood that an individual might die within a certain period. Graunt and Petty had called for the assemblage of an historical record so that questions about current and future mortality, and about population trend, might be answered. The techniques they brought to bear were useful also to the environmentalist, who had to discover relative frequencies before he could find associations between environment and disease. It cannot be said that mathematical expectation was quickly mastered in an age of low numeracy. But the procedure – an adaptation from a technique familiar in commerce for making exchange calculations – [12] provided those who could use it with a means to infer unknowns (the probable size of a lottery prize, or the future mortality rate) from knowns (the total tickets, prize-winning tickets, and prizes, or historic mortality and population). And if only a few physicians in the eighteenth century explicitly applied this formula to their inquiries, nevertheless the results reported by those who did use it entered discourse about disease and the environment. Furthermore, the entire procedure of discovering ratios of phenomena and using those to project trend, which was common in the eighteenth century,[13] is an application of mathematical expectation, even if the ratio-maker did not realise that.

From the first, the medicine of the environment drew on the new political arithmetic of Graunt and Petty. The habitat was to be observed in any event, but especially whenever observations could be given quantitative expression, such as in mortality and morbidity statistics, and measures of rainfall, elevation, barometric pressure, and temperature. Application of the fundamental techniques of statistical inquiry, of procedures that stepped beyond the mere aggregation of cases, occurred in medicine for the first time in a systematic fashion in the medicine of the environment.

In meteorology, too, the seventeenth century was a period of innovations, of which some contributed directly to the environmentalist's search for a technique for characterising and quantifying features of the environment. During that century the instruments necessary to measure temperature, atmospheric pressure, wind velocity, humidity, rainfall, and other traits of climate and weather were invented or improved.[14] At the end of the century these instruments remained, in most cases, inaccurate (or unreliably accurate), and the techniques employed in their use (such as taking temperature readings at different times of the day, or inside and outside a dwelling) imperfect. As late as 1800 the distinction between atmospheric and relative humidity remained unclear.[15] This is a particularly important ambiguity, for the environmentalists took humidity to be one of the most significant features of weather and climate. Nevertheless physicians used these instruments and data gathered from them to build a quantitative picture of weather and climate.

The practice of regularly recording observations of weather phenomena emerged toward the middle of the seventeenth century. In following decades manuals describing how to build and use meteorological instruments appeared,[16] and the practice of recording daily readings of temperature, barometric pressure, wind force and direction and general weather conditions spread rapidly. A vague but sweeping notion about the ultimate usefulness of such records guided the effort. In the *Philosophical Transactions* of 1666, the physicist and chemist Robert Boyle published a paper on the collection of meteorological observations, arguing that the weather in a locale could be linked both to epidemics and to the general salubrity of the air (that is, the climate).[17] In the eighteenth century this interest in gathering meteorological readings gained momentum. The learned periodicals of Europe and North America frequently printed weather and climate data, and many people – inspired by the feeling that a long enough series of records would be revealing – kept private journals. These observations of the environment furnished the physician with a vast body of data. Since general morbidity and specific diseases waxed and waned with the seasons and changes in the weather, these records seemed also to contain the as yet unsorted secret of the manner in which weather and climate influence sickness and health.

The Enlightenment View of Nature

Another seventeenth-century contribution to environmentalist thought is to be found in what Clarence Glacken refers to as the first steps toward the 'breathtaking anthropocentrism' of twentieth-century man, steps that lie in the rise of a conviction of control over nature.[18] Sometimes in the past seen as a benign, and at other times as a malevolent force, nature came in the seventeenth century to be viewed as an object for manipulation. This theme figures prominently in population theory, where a branch of thinkers designated physico-theologians seemed to have discovered both a divine plan for population and, in the hands of the Lutheran cleric Süssmilch, ways to modify man and nature to make them conform more closely to this plan.[19] This development is still better known as a feature of thought in the physical sciences, and in the late seventeenth-century image of a universal mechanism resembling a clock. It arose, Glacken maintains, from the seventeenth-century contact of science and technology, from the integration into scientific thought of the notion that man was successfully controlling some features of nature (such as in Dutch polder-building). In believing that man's habitat might be modified to render it healthier, the environmentalist shared with many others – Descartes, Derham, Nieuwentijd, Süssmilch, and Bacon, to mention only a few names – a new sense that man's surroundings might be modified and managed. This 'idea of man as a finisher of nature, a completer of the creation' both arises from and leads to religious and secular conclusions.[20] This short list of names, which includes both secular and religious thinkers, illustrates the point. In short, this feature of the origins of the medicine of the environment does not attach physicians any more closely to the scientific revolution than it attaches them to the late seventeenth- and eighteenth-century attempt to find an explanation for new scientific discoveries consonant with traditional religious belief. It merely links them to the eighteenth-century effort to improve man's surroundings, to find those panaceas that would promote happiness.[21]

Environmentalism is therefore not a branch of medicine that can be detached from seventeenth- and eighteenth-century thought in general. It is rather a branch in which physicians shared with other thinkers both a more intense interest in nature and an expectation about human potential. Nature seemed to constitute a great harmony. Yet man lived in discord with this harmony, one sign of which lay in the prevalence of epidemic disease. What struck medical and non-medical observers alike was man's failure yet to discover all those measures that would end discord, and man's failure to adopt and abide by those things that were known. To notice this is to notice that physicians drew upon influences outside medicine, and that medicine, insofar as it adopted this view of man and nature, contributed its own part to the eighteenth-century development toward the breathtaking anthropocentrism of the twentieth century. Let us look with particular care at the timing of the Enlightenment shift from thought to action, from reflection about the problems of man to action to redress those problems. This shift can be dated to the 1740s and 1750s,[22] which is also the period in which we will discover a shift in the medicine of the environment from thought to action. This is not a coincidence. This phase of the Enlightenment both inspired and drew inspiration from environmentalism.

ENVIRONMENTAL PATHOLOGY IN ITS FIRST PHASE

In the sense of direct and immediate origins, the medicine of the environment emerged in the work of a group of English and Anglo-Irish physicians and physicists during the period from the 1660s–80s. In those years Robert Boyle, Robert Hooke, William Petty, John Locke, Christopher Wren, and Thomas Sydenham introduced two streams of inquiry into the study of disease.[23] The physicians among them would examine the nature of disease through clinical observation and case histories. This stream would lead to an improved classification, the objective of which was to help distinguish successful methods of treatment. These physicians and the physicists also would study in addition the 'constitution' of disease (especially epidemic disease) by examining the milieu of disease and the intersection of environmental features coinciding with epidemics. This stream would, it seemed likely, lead to an improved understanding of the causes of disease.

Eighteenth-century physicians tended to assume that these inquiries – especially those of Sydenham, who gathered case histories of diseases and weather – had produced a coherent version of the content, methods, and aims of environmental pathology. In fact such a coherent statement may first be found in a book that the satirist, mathematician, and physician John Arbuthnot published in 1733 under the title *An Essay Concerning the Effects of Air on Human Bodies*. Attributing much to Sydenham, Arbuthnot offered a general theory, the elements of which he extracted from the work of English and Irish predecessors and from the writings of continental physicians. The first phase of the medicine of the environment, which lasted from the 1660s until 1733, was a phase in which many explanations of disease causation were considered before a few were isolated for intensive investigation.

Sydenham's interests, we have already seen, mirror this generalised search for a more efficacious medicine. When therefore Boyle endorsed the idea that a cause of epidemic disease might be found in emanations from the earth and diseased persons (in Boyle's view, specifically inorganic subterranean corpuscular or particulate emanations mixed with other atmospheric elements),[24] Sydenham was only mildly interested. Whereas he accepted environmental variables as causes of disease, he did not wish to focus on them.[25] It is nevertheless this conjuncture of ideas that seems to fashion the beginning of the new medicine of the environment. From Boyle's affirmation of an idea taken from classical Greek medicine, and from Sydenham's warm if rather succinct approval of it grew the notion that an improved theory of disease causation could be built upon intensive study of weather, climate, milieu, and mortality.[26] The experimentation of Hooke and Wren with meteorological instruments, Locke's daily weather records (kept off and on for nearly forty years), Locke's and Boyle's published meteorological observations,[27] and Petty's study of mortality and mortality records responded to an expectation that, by counting and measuring certain traits of man and his environment, it would be possible to discover the rules believed to govern the relationship between disease and these other variables. By observing and recording the prevailing epidemic fevers according to the season of the year and the meteorological signs under which they occurred, one could infer which environmental complex caused which epidemic.

In Sydenham's hands it was not a quantitative but a qualitative record from which understanding of the epidemic constitution would be sought. A chronicle of London's large-group diseases during 1661–75 revealed to him five distinct constitutions, for instance the dysenteric constitution of 1670–2.[28] Each could be supposed to be associated with the season of the year and other factors. But, as we know already, Sydenham was less concerned to record the features of atmospheric or environmental constitutions than he was to describe the epidemic constitution and summarise his clinical findings. Although he affirmed Boyle's idea about emanations, he professed to find the operation of that force often inscrutable.[29] As D. G. Bates explains, Sydenham compiled epidemic histories in search of understanding of an unknown force, an *X* factor, in causation.[30] Certain atmospheric and environmental complexes seemed to operate regularly and predictably in producing certain epidemics. But Sydenham noticed that others functioned so unpredictably that a cure useful for a certain disease at one time might be positively harmful in the same disease at another time.[31]

Still Sydenham, like Hippocrates, identified five phenomena worthy of close attention: heat, cold, moisture, dryness, and emanations (from the earth and from pathological matter, whether human, animal, or inanimate).[32] Of these the first four were seen, with season, to comprise the chief forces behind an atmospheric constitution, and the fifth the chief elements of an environmental constitution. Sydenham also hazarded that breathing constitutes the primary method of infection – that is, that the inhalation of elements from the atmospheric and environmental constitution brings on disease. Later environmentalists would broaden this list of elements within the atmospheric and environmental constitutions and expand the designation of means of transmission. But they would adhere closely to Sydenham's sense of the mechanism at work, and to his style of reporting on epidemic constitutions. More than a century later, Louis Lépecq de La Clôture described the disease constitutions of Normandy during 1763–77 in a form similar to that used by Sydenham, although with considerably more detail.[33]

More specifically, Sydenham attributed certain diseases (among them plague) chiefly to the environmental constitution, and others (such as intermittent fevers and pleurisy) to the atmospheric constitution, and a third group (e.g., gout) to humoural imbalance. He also distinguished certain diseases termed stationary fevers (the prevailing diseases of certain periods) from another category, intercurrent fevers, in such a fashion as to suggest that a given epidemic might be influenced not merely by environmental factors but also by other large-group diseases of the same period. Rather ambiguously Sydenham thus fashioned the idea of a morbidity complex – an overlapping of diseases – as a way of accounting for what could not otherwise be accounted for within his system, and for explaining the need for a sensitive approach to therapies.

Still, it was upon the reigning diseases that he concentrated. The stationary fevers, he wrote, 'depend upon some particular, but hitherto undiscovered, condition of the constitution of the particular year'. The intercurrent fevers – rheumatism, scarlet fever, and pleurisy, among others – while still epidemic in their occurrence, may 'originate in some particular anomaly of some particular bodies' or be 'due to some general atmospheric influence'.[34] For instance, sudden temperature changes in spring cause pleurisy. Sydenham distinguished such causes from the causes providing the occasion for individual cases of intercurrent or stationary fevers, but he did not try to define a boundary between large-group and individual manifestations of disease. Even if some uncertainty remained about disease causation, Sydenham believed without reservation in the efficacy of one or another mix of certain remedies, chiefly bleeding, sweating, purging, and some drug compounds.[35]

After Sydenham's death a myth developed about the power and clarity of his ideas. John Locke advanced that myth by consistently praising Sydenham, even though the two men had disagreed on a number of issues, such as the utility of purges or the gathering of abundant meteorological observations. With Charles Goodall, Locke furthered Sydenham's reputation by asking, in a questionnaire sent to physicians outside Britain, about 'the esteeme which Phisitians have had of Doctor Sydenham and his works'.[36] When eighteenth-century physicians cited a mythical view of Sydenham's achievements to justify their own environmentalist ideas, they thus affirmed the power of a carefully cultivated effort to build Sydenham's reputation.

Boyle's contribution to this theory lay in two large areas. First, he investigated the properties of the atmosphere, thereby directing attention toward the air as an interesting realm of scientific inquiry. Fascination with pneumatic chemistry would wax and wane during the eighteenth century, but throughout would prevail the assumption that decomposition of the properties of the air must contribute to understanding of the diseases caused, transmitted, or influenced by it. Second, Boyle formulated a corpuscular philosophy which he applied to several areas of research. In pneumatic chemistry the theory of an atmosphere composed of and holding in suspension minute particles seemed to identify the agents of causation or transmission of disease, so that Boyle furnished environmentalism with something concrete – albeit still largely hypothetical – to investigate. As the renowned French physician Boissier de Sauvages explained in 1754 in a general account of the theory of the atmosphere as a reservoir of disease, the air is composed of homogeneous molecules, but it also contains heterogeneous particles, some of which are impure or unhealthy.[37] In environmental pathology the corpuscular theory of the atmosphere formed part of the means of accounting for how air influences disease, the other part being the meteorological qualities of the air, such as temperature and barometric pressure.

One of the characteristics of this theory was that it was vague, for Boyle's corpuscules merged with the miasmas of Hippocratic tradition so that some environmentalists wrote indeterminately about exhalations and emanations. Often it is not clear whether they meant to refer to physical matter, although it is rare indeed to find any overt suggestion of ethereal forms. One physician, L. S. D. Le Brun of Meaux, complained of the indiscriminate use of a variety of imprecise terms – leaven, virus, miasmas, morbific molecules, and contagious corpuscules – to describe the exhalations of sick individuals.[38] In fact eighteenth-century writers used the word 'miasma' to mean both vaporous exhalations (for example, as associated with the stench of putrefying organic matter) and particles suspended in the atmosphere. These usages seem to anticipate the modern theory of droplet nuclei, pathogenic particles light enough to remain suspended in the air for considerable periods. Eighteenth-century commentators believed both vapours and particles to be harmful, or potentially harmful, to community health.[39] Over the course of the century less attention fell on the form of these things and more on their varieties. Noël Retz explained that 'the elements that are exhaled in abundance from the soil, the waters, and from different substances, and which are suspended in the air, being susceptible to an infinite number of combinations, can be expected to produce results equally varied'.[40] A multiplicity of particulate and vaporous matter thus joined a numerous variety of meteorological phenomena, together to fashion an explanation for the causes of disease.

Not all notions linking disease to the habitat came to be incorporated in the medicine of the environment, and one that was not incorporated is climatic determinism. Already by the 1660s interest in Hippocratic ideas about milieu and disease had a long, if sporadic, history.[41] In some early natural histories of the New World, for example Willem Piso's account of Brazil, there are elements strongly suggestive of medical topography. In a similar vein continental physicians had, at least since the fifteenth century, explored links between occupation and disease. But if there is at all a continuous stream in attentiveness to this part of the Hippocratic tradition, that stream lay not in linking disease to the milieu but in accounting for character and temperament by means of climate. Sydenham's contemporary, John Goad, reaffirmed this tradition in a 1686 book entitled *Astro-meteorologica, or Aphorisms and Discourses of the Bodies Celestial.* Mixing astrology and weather descriptions, Goad claimed to explain how climate and weather affect temperament and disposition. These kinds of arguments would continue to be made in the eighteenth century, such as in the abbé Dubos' case for a climatic determination of artistic talent,[42] and Montesquieu's general theory of climatic influence. Nevertheless environmentalists did not attach much weight to such assumptions.

Some part of the explanation for this neglect may lie in the controversial nature of climatic determinism. In a 1748 essay, 'Of National Characters', David Hume doubted 'that men owe any thing of their temper or genius to the air, food, or climate', (although he did not deny the existence of national character: 'An ENGLISHMAN will naturally be supposed to have more knowledge than a DANE').[43] A more general reason for the environmentalists' shift away from the kind of arguments made by Goad is to be found in the undifferentiated nature of the links supposed to exist between climate and temperament or character. The matters to which Goad pointed could not be defined even as well as the sometimes still vague associations identified by Sydenham. What is more, they defied measurement. And, finally, later passages will reveal the cosmopolitan quality of environmentalism, and the extent to which environmentalists in many countries read one another's books and essays. Clearly they knew that disease is inattentive to political and linguistic boundaries, and they could detect more variations in climate in Europe than in the range of common epidemic diseases.

Sources of Disease

How did the early environmentalists work out the problem of explaining the sources of disease? We know, from what has already been said, that the medicine of the environment was more conventional than unconventional in its use of sources, that Sydenham and his associates and followers were more comfortable with the familiar than the unfamiliar. They offered not a departure from, but a variation on, existing ideas about aetiology.[44] These ideas found their sources in either humoural pathology or in a contagion theory sometimes hinting at the existence of microorganisms (in a manner analogous to Boyle's hints toward the suspension of pathogenic matter in the air). In humoural pathology, which itself underlay classical notions about the influence of climate on human health and character,[45] the capacity for or the seeds of disease or pain was believed to lie within the body awaiting release. Release might occur as the result of diet, physical activity, or contact with other external agents, such as weather in certain forms or sequences. All these forces could, it was believed, be controlled (or at least influenced) by the prescription of appropriate health regimens, purges, diaphoresis, and sometimes bleeding.

In environmental pathology, in contrast, air remained an external agent capable of provoking disease, but the role assigned to it was both altered and shifted in emphasis. In the early theory, as elaborated by Sydenham, air served still as a catalytic force, provoking the internal bodily humours into disharmony, but operating more forcefully than was traditionally allowed in humoural pathology. Later, as more distinct environmentalist theory of disease aetiology developed, the air came to be seen as being by itself a sufficient cause of disease. By

Arbuthnot's day the entirely consistent environmentalist no longer needed to hypothesise about humoural imbalance because the intermediary role of the humours had been eliminated as a causal factor behind epidemics. The air was no longer one among six non-naturals[46] – influences external to the body seen in classical medicine as causes of health and (if abused) of disease – but instead the primary agent of disease. As Arbuthnot explained, the environmentalist should seek to identify the 'nosopoerick' qualities of the atmosphere, that is, those qualities with 'a Power of producing Diseases'.[47] Environmentalism retained the non-naturals as a means of explaining certain aspects of individual and large-group disease and their avoidance. But it vastly changed the significance attached to the first of them – air.

What made an environmentalist explanation of epidemic causation seem more persuasive than a humoural explanation was the very difficulty of using a single theory to account for both individual and epidemic cases of disease. Sydenham explained that sporadic cases of the plague, for example, could be assumed to be uninfluenced by the atmospheric or environmental constitution, and to be produced instead by contagion.[48] It is only epidemics that are caused by an atmospheric or environmental constitution. As a means of accounting for large-group disease, the sixteenth-century contagion theory seemed, by the late seventeenth and early eighteenth century, unpersuasive. This theory, identified especially with Girolamo Fracastoro, explained epidemics by referring to minute infective agents or spores transmitted directly from person to person, indirectly via intermediaries, and through the air.[49] These agents, he believed, 'acted on the humours and vital spirits of the body'.[50] Environmentalists did not discard these ideas. In some diseases, primarily smallpox and measles, contagion continued to be cited to explain the onset of an epidemic. In other diseases, such as yellow fever, contagion was sometimes allowed to take over once the disease had appeared.[51] But the substance of contagion was often one or another of the agents identified in environmentalist theory as causes of epidemics. Boyle's corpuscular theory incorporated the idea of particulate elements of contagion.

In short, no distinct boundary between the contagion theory of the sixteenth century and the environmentalist theory of the eighteenth century can be discovered because the two theories overlapped. What is more, distinctive elements of the two theories were left obscure in the eighteenth century by the environmentalists' modification and subsummation of contagion theory. Clifton Wintringham, a leading figure in the second generation of British environmentalists, explained how contagion should be construed. There are, on the one hand, endemic diseases, and on the other epidemic diseases. 'Endemic Diseases . . . owe their Origin to some particular Qualities of the Climate, Air, Soil, Situation, Waters, and the like'.[52] 'Contagious Diseases [e.g., smallpox and most fevers]. . . are capable of being communicated to us by the Air, or the Effluvia of morbid Bodies'.[53] 'The Causes therefore of these Diseases must either be generated in the Air, or produced from the Effluvia of animal, vegetable, or mineral Substances floating in it'.[54] In the tradition of Sydenham, therefore, the environment was construed to be both the remote cause for the appearance of epidemics and the agency of their transmission.[55]

But why were environmentalist ideas accounted more persuasive than traditional contagionist explanations of epidemic and endemic disease? This question was considered by Arbuthnot, like Sydenham, chiefly in terms of the comparatively well documented case of the bubonic plague. The old contagion theory and its 'invisible Insects' or inanimate infection agents may sometimes explain the causes of epidemics,[56] but they are not a sufficient explanation. This is so because the plague has been observed to occur at much the same time in widely separate locales that are not known to have had any contact with one another. Only a universal cause can account for such a thing. As universal cause Arbuthnot proposed 'the Hypothesis of extraordinary Effluvia' – that is, Boyle's emanations – according to which any locale is susceptible to any constitution of the atmosphere and thus to any disease.[57] 'I think one may conclude, That the Constitution of the Air is the chief Instrument perhaps in producing, but surely in propagating and extinguishing this Distemper'.[58] To Arbuthnot the effluvia could be either particulate or vaporous. He cited an explanation for the origin of the plague of 1346. It began in the Kingdom of Cathay in a 'vapour most horridly foetid, that breaking out of the Earth, like a kind of subterraneal Fire, consumed and destroyed above 200 Leagues of that Country. . . and infected the Air'. Then it was transmitted to Greece and the rest of Europe.[59]

What is more, the periodic change of the atmospheric constitution – either with the seasons alone or jointly with other forces – seemed to explain the seasonal flux of disease. In contrast, the contagion theory as then understood failed because it lacked a sense of the potential for exhaustion of the factors conducive to the survival and spread of microorganisms. Even the theorists who attributed a large role in plague aetiology to contagion, as did Richard Mead, assigned to atmospheric conditions the capacity to aid or hinder propagation of the disease in a determinant fashion. Mead thus accounted for the conclusion of plague epidemics by means of a change in the atmospheric constitution, in which, for instance, weather conditions might halt an epidemic.[60] In this way, the contagion theory was revised to take on some of the aspects of environmentalism.

Arbuthnot thus joined Boyle and Sydenham, contagion and environmentalist theory. By asserting a doctrine of effluvia, Arbuthnot held that emanations from the earth may combine with atmospheric or meteorological properties and qualities to cause epidemics. If in a particular case these were not the cause, then emanations from diseased persons or from other sources could be assumed to have entered the environmental constitution, transforming a single or a few cases of illness into an epidemic.[61] Here Arbuthnot agreed with some elements of a case made in 1717 by the Roman physician Giovanni Lancisi about the origins of malaria.[62] Lancisi held to the operation of two means by which swamps produce malaria, one partially animate (in which visible insects, mosquitoes, carry pathogenic matter in the form of fluids) and another inanimate (in which swamp emanations infect the atmosphere). In other words, Lancisi, who sketched a map of marshes and wind directions,[63] adhered simultaneously to the old contagion theory and to the environmentalist theory. But it was principally his theory of swamp emanations that caught the attention of eighteenth-century readers, who counted Lancisi as one of the major early spokesmen of environmentalist theory.

The feature that made the mature form of environmentalist theory so attractive was its absorption of the principal element of contagion theory. Not only emanations from earth but also emanations from diseased people, corpses, rotting vegetable matter, and other sources might add to the atmospheric constitution the properties and qualities necessary to provoke an epidemic. In the nineteenth century these emanations were usually construed to be vapours rather than organic or inorganic matter, and it is in that form that we are familiar with them in our pejorative assessment of miasmic theory. We have noticed, however, that in early environmentalist theory the emanations were many things, including vapours.

One implication of the environmentalist shift in thinking must be singled out for notice. The conventional notion of the quarantine, which asserted the contagious nature of disease, conflicted in some respects with environmentalist assumptions. The physician of the milieu turned this idea on its head, applying it not to the isolation of the already diseased from the still healthy, but to the isolation of the still healthy from the site of disease, and from the epidemic constitution. One of this physician's objectives was to devise a plan of disease avoidance by means of quarantining or modifying the pathogenic site.

ARBUTHNOT ON METHOD

Locke, Petty, and Sydenham gathered data on, respectively, weather and climate, mortality, and epidemic constitutions. They thus showed those who would follow them what specifically to do to develop environmentalist theory. They inspired other physicians to compile epidemic histories, meteorological journals, and mortality registers, and to report their findings in books and learned journals in the expectation that, once the data series had been compared with one another, the comparison would reveal the associations provoking epidemics. In York, Clifton Wintringham kept a record of epidemics and meteorological phenomena during 1715–25.[64] John Huxham, a Plymouth physician known for his work on classifying fevers, similarly began his own record of the same phenomena in 1724.[65] In recording meteorological observations, he followed the form set forth by James Jurin in a 1723 article in the *Philosophical Transactions*.[66] Huxham also took care to describe his instruments, a matter of considerable importance because of the growing variety of meteorological tools and systems of measurement. Patrick Ker compared meteorological and disease experience among four sites (Edinburgh, Ripon, Plymouth, and Nürnberg), searching for an international verification of the theory and a demonstration that adjustments might be made for variable meteorological readings from different instruments.[67] In this way a substantial historical record of environmental and pathological evidence began to accumulate, some of it in print and some in manuscript.

John Arbuthnot, a Scot and in Dr. Johnson's phrase 'the most universal genius' knew something of this compilation of evidence by British and continental physicians. He had also taken the trouble to read the more theoretical literature on disease. He intended in his 1733 book to bring thought and action together. But with Arbuthnot we must beware of a fine taste in humour. Friend of Pope and Swift and, with them, a member of the Scriblerus Club, Arbuthnot is more often remembered for his wit and satire – for instance in using the character John Bull to typify the traits of Englishmen – than for his contributions to medicine or mathematics. But he could be serious, as he proved by translating Huygens' text on mathematical expectation and probability theory into English.[68] In an intriguing life Arbuthnot served twice as physician to the Queen, cared for a time for a wild boy named Peter found wandering in the woods of Hamlen in Hanover and brought to England in 1725, wrote knowledgeably on the history of weights and measures, and in an 'Essay on the Usefulness of Mathematical Learning' sought to stimulate the teaching and use of mathematics in physics and medicine.[69] Arbuthnot's *An Essay Concerning the Effects of Air on Human Bodies*,[70] and its companion, a 1731 treatise on alimentation and health, were entirely serious.

In this formative discourse on environmental pathology Arbuthnot summarised the substantial number of ideas already in circulation, and tied them to the researches of Edmund Halley and Stephen Hales, among others, into the properties of air. Two years previously Hales had argued that the operation of plant life varied according to temperature and humidity,[71] which constituted an analogy adding force to the notion that such climatic forces influence man in obvious and subtle ways. To these ideas Arbuthnot added inferences drawn from his own medical practice, which stretched back to 1696. Restating the notion that disease, especially epidemic disease, may be accounted for by the prevailing environmental constitution, he sought to specify which elements of that constitution were operative in individual epidemics, and to identify research steps that might verify features of the environmental hypothesis. Certain research programs executed for a long enough period would 'perhaps reduce the Physiology of the Air to a Science' in itself.[72]

Arbuthnot wished also to catalogue inferences about the environment and disease, to which end he listed a hundred aphorisms drawn from his own inferences, Hippocratic writings, and an otherwise unidentified epidemic history of Germany.[73] In his formulation of a theory of environmental pathology Arbuthnot had little to say that was new. But the ideas behind this emerging branch of medical inquiry had nowhere before either been explained so fully or stated so coherently as an independent system of thought. For those reasons (and because of the large influence that Arbuthnot had on the later development of environmentalism),[74] this essay deserves consideration in still more detail. For the moment let us store up some insights and assumptions from the medicine of the environment; their significance will emerge later.

Whereas his predecessors had begun their excursions into the idea of epidemic constitutions by examining epidemics, Arbuthnot began by looking at the atmosphere. The earth's atmosphere is a single entity, he explained, and it is fluid. The air in one place is constantly changing. If this fluidity is interfered with, such as by shutting people up in an area closed to circulation, then the ordinarily healthy atmosphere will become noxious, as Hales demonstrated in experiments on the respiration of animals confined to closed quarters. Although in general the atmosphere is fluid and constantly in motion, the air of any given location possesses a particular mixture of additives and influences which give it its environmental constitution. These additives and influences Arbuthnot termed 'properties' and 'qualities'. Among the properties, atmospheric pressure will vary from time to time and place to place, and the pressure at one time and place will compose one element of the environmental constitution of that time and place. These properties (atmospheric pressure, air density, fluidity, and others) Arbuthnot added to the elements that Sydenham had identified (heat, cold, moisture and dryness). Following classical Greek precedent, Arbuthnot termed these four things qualities of the air.[75] Each quality makes its own contribution to the atmospheric constitution. 'Air, by the Properties and Qualities enumerated, must produce very sensible changes in Human Bodies, because it not only operates by outward Contact, but we constantly imbibe it at all the Pores of the Body'. To Sydenham's more restricted idea about the means of infection (breathing), Arbuthnot thus added the more insidious notion of mere contact: 'Nothing accounts more clearly for epidemical Diseases seizing Human Creatures inhabiting the same Tract of Earth, who have nothing in common that affects them, except Air'.[76]

Arbuthnot explained further that, in addition to these properties and qualities, the environmental constitution of a given place and time will be shaped by emanations from the earth and waters of that site. Whereas the properties and qualities of the air are found generally in the atmosphere and are always changing, local emanations are specific and constant. It is the mutual influence of the two types of forces that explains why certain epidemics prevail in certain locales, and why the same epidemic may be found in regions far distant from one another which have not had any known contact. The theory of environmentalism thus resolved the great puzzle of contagion theory.

Arbuthnot also identified certain things worthy of attention and measurement. To Sydenham's short list of temperature and humidity he added atmospheric pressure. In place of the unspecific reference to emanations, Arbuthnot pointed to such specific phenomena as the saline and mineral content of dew, which could be measured by chemical analysis.[77] He thus lengthened the list of phenomena of which measurements needed to be made and histories kept during the long era of data collection that would verify or refine things already known (or presumed) about the environment–disease association. In its present state the theory of epidemic constitutions was, Arbuthnot held, 'almost Scientific'.[78] It would be made fully scientific when the necessary records had been accumulated and, like nosologies built from the case histories of individual patients, those had been reduced to a system specifying associations. From 'Journals of the Weather, Reigning Diseases, and Remedies successful . . . perhaps it might be possible to predict both the Weather and the epidemic Diseases'.[79] Quite obviously Arbuthnot believed the hurdle of reconceptualising the causes of epidemic disease to have been surmounted. His own task was to point out the lane to be followed to make the theory functional. In a phrase, Arbuthnot felt comfortable in drawing conclusions at this early stage of data collection.

To illustrate the methodology of environmentalism, and perhaps also to authenticate it from experience, Arbuthnot cited the case of the catarrhal fever (influenza) epidemic of late 1732 and early 1733.[80] It was, he believed, an epidemic of general and perhaps nearly universal occurrence over the globe.[81] Some patience will be required to read this rather long description. The reward will take two forms: 1) we shall see directly into the thinking of an environmentalist, and learn more about why the environment–disease association seemed so persuasive; and 2) we shall learn something about a low fatality epidemic, a common event which is often overlooked in disease histories for the sake of heavily fatal epidemics, and we shall thereby take a step toward specifying and refining Sydenham's idea of a morbidity complex.

> The previous Constitution of the Air was, in *England*, and in the greatest Part of *Europe*, a great Drought, which may be inferr'd from the Failure of the Springs, in the Abatement of the fresh Water in all its usual Currents and Reservoirs, which are the best Measure of the Quantity of Moisture falling from the Clouds. What is most generally taken notice of in the Accounts I have seen from *Germany*, *France*, and some other Places, was, That the Air in the beginning of Winter, especially in *November*, was more than usually filled with thick and frequent Fogs, the Matter of which was not precipitated upon the Earth in Rain, Snow, or any other Fruits of the Air. Fogs are so usual in this Country in *November*, that there was nothing particular observ'd about them that I know. But there was hardly any thing fell from the Clouds during the Month of *November*, except a very small Quantity of Snow, attended with a Frost of no long Duration; and this was all the Winter we had. In the Northern Parts of *France* there was a very small Quantity of Snow, which lasted from their 15th and our 4th of *November*, till after *Christmas*. This was succeeded by Southerly Winds and stinking Fogs, during which there was observ'd by some Chirurgeons a great Disposition in Wounds to mortify. Both before and during the Continuance of the Disease in *England*, the Air was warm, beyond the usual Temper of the Season, with great Quantities of sulphureous Vapours, producing great Storms of Wind from the South-West, and sometimes Lightning without Thunder.

As to the Time of Invasion of the Disease, they were different in different countries. It invaded *Saxony* and the neighbouring Countries in Germany, about the 15th of *November*, and lasted in its Vigour till the 29th of the same Month. It was earlier in *Holland* than in *England*; earlier in *Edinburg* than in *London*. It was in *New England* before it attack'd *Britain*; in *London*, before it reach'd some other Places westward, as *Oxford*, *Bath*, &c. and, as far as I can collect from Accounts, it invaded the Northerly Parts of *Europe* before the Southerly. It lasted in its Vigour in *London*, from about the middle of *January* 1732/3, for about 3 Weeks; the Bill of Mortality, from *Tuesday* the 23d to *Tuesday* the 30th of *January*, contain'd in all 1588, being higher than any time since the Plague. It began in *Paris* about the beginning of their *February*, or the 21st of our *January*, and lasted till the beginning of their *April*, or the 21st of our *March*; and I think its Duration was longest in the southerly Countries. It raged in *Naples* and the southern Parts of *Italy* in our *March*. The Disease, in traveling from Place to Place, did not observe the Direction, but went often contrary to the Course of the Winds.

The Uniformity of the Symptoms of the Disease in every Place was most remarkable. A small Rigor or Chilliness, succeeded with a Fever of a Duration (in such as recover'd) seldom above three Days. This Fever was attended with a Headache, sometimes Pains in the Back, Thirst in no great Degree, a Catarrh or thin Defluxion, occasioning Sneezing; a *Coryza*, or Running at the Nose; a Cough with Expectoration of a thin Pituite at first, and afterwards of a viscous Matter; in which, if there was observ'd a clear oily Matter, it prov'd generally the Case to be mortal, for this clear Matter was purulent. These were the most common Symptoms: But a great many during that Season were affected with Spitting of Blood, Pleurisies, and Inflammations of the Lungs, dangerous, and often mortal; in some Places, particularly in *France*, the Fever after six or seven Days ended in miliary Eruptions; in *Holland* often in Imposthumations of the Throat; in all the Blood was sizy; and every where the Disease was particularly fatal to aged People. What was observable was, that the Fever left a Debility and Dejection of Appetite and Spirits, much more than in Proportion to its Strength or Duration; and the

Cough outlasted the Fever is some more than six Weeks or two Months.

There was during the whole Season, a great Run of Hysterical, Hypochondriacal, and Nervous Distempers; in short, all the Symptoms of Relaxation. These Symptoms were so high in some as to produce a sort of Fatuity or Madness, in which, for some Hours together, they would be seiz'd with a wandering of their Senses, mistaking their common Affairs; at the same time they had not any great Degree or a Fever to confine them to their Beds; but in several who were thus affected, the Urine was observ'd often to change from pale to turbid, alternately, so that there was some Fever, tho' I did not observe nor hear that the Bark was effectual, but the saline Febrifuge Draughts had generally a most surprising good Effect. Since this Disease has been over, the Air has continued to be particularly noxious in Diseases which affect the Lungs, and for that Reason occasioning a great and unusual Mortality of the Meazles, at the Rate of 40 in a Week, from which one has reason to expect some specialities in the Diseases of the succeeding Season.

The Remedies commonly successful in this epidemical catarrhous Fever were Bleeding, Sweating, promoted by watery Diaphoreticks, Blisters, and the common pectoral Medicines; and what I observ'd before, Febrifuge Draughts of Salt, of Wormwood, Juice of Limon, *&c.* I have not Particulars enough to enable me to enter into the Aetiology of this Distemper.

It was Matter of Fact that there was a previous ill Constitution of the Air, noxious to animal Bodies. In *Autumn*, and long afterwards, a Madness among Dogs; the Horses were seiz'd with the Catarrh before Mankind; and a Gentleman averr'd to me, that some Birds, particularly the Sparrows, left the Place where he was during the Sickness.

The previous great Drought, as has been observ'd before, must have been particularly hurtful to Mankind: Great Droughts exert their Effects after the Surface of the Earth is again opened by Moisture; and the Perspiration of the Ground, which was long suppress'd, is suddenly restor'd. It is probable that the Earth then emits several new Effluvia hurtful to Human Bodies; that this appear'd to be the Case by the thick

> and stinking Fogs which succeeded the Rain that had fall'n before.
>
> It is likewise evident that these Effluvia were not of any particular or mineral Nature, because they were of a Substance that was common to every Part of the Surface of the Earth; and therefore one may conclude that they were watery Exhalations, or at least such mix'd with other exhalable Substances that are common to every Spot of Ground.
>
> Lastly, It is agreeable to Experience that watery Effluvia are hurtful to the Glands of the Windpipe and the Lungs, and productive of Catarrhs.

In short, this in London during one week the most severe of all epidemics since the plague arose from an environmental complex of drought, certain kinds of fogs, unseasonably high temperatures, sulphurous vapours, and wind storms from the southwest. Its coming was forecast by certain responses among animals. In retrospect some remedies and treatments seemed to have been more effective than others. We will not be impressed by Arbuthnot's logic or hopeful about his preferred remedies. It is not important that we should accept the environmentalist's arguments and inferences, but that we should see what they were. Later we shall inquire more carefully into why these arguments were accounted persuasive. And later still we shall investigate what the environmentalists proposed to do to remove, or avoid, the problem of pathogenic habitats. In the meantime, we must shift our attention from John Arbuthnot, who died in February 1735, to another Scottish physician, Thomas Short, who around 1731 began a programme of data collection.

THOMAS SHORT

In 1733 Arbuthnot could cite a few sources containing weather journals and disease histories of the sort providing the raw data needed to build a physiology of the air and a medicine of climates and places. He could point also to a larger array of sources containing sporadic observations of some use. He could, for example, mention Hans Sloane's Jamaican journal and Ramazzini's Modena records on 1690–4, and he could use the numerous travel accounts of that era as a source. But the comprehensive and systematic record-keeping that Arbuthnot advised had not yet been executed. Something of that sort was, however, under way. In Sheffield Thomas Short had begun, some two years earlier, a programme of observations that he would sustain for nearly twenty years and report upon in books published in 1747 and 1750. Whereas Arbuthnot sketched out the first modern general theory of environmentalism, Short sought to develop the first full and systematic repertoire of associations between the environment and epidemic disease. As recently as 1948 the medical statistician and epidemiologist Major Greenwood could suggest that Short's conclusions about the influence of locale upon salubrity 'are now part of the common stock of lay and, perhaps, professional belief'.[82] Like Arbuthnot, Short relied not merely on his own observations but also on the collective wisdom of his day. His was *A General Chronological History of the Air, Weather, Seasons, Meteors, &c. in Sundry Places and Different Times; More Particularly for the Space of 250 Years*.[83]

But what should be observed? To Arbuthnot's longer list of variables Short added still more potentially influential factors and forces, and extended the investigation beyond the issue of environmental medicine. Asking 'what Soils, Situations, Trades, Manners of Life, &c. are best adapted to Health and Long Life', he considered, or urged that someone consider: age, sex, physical makeup, season of the year, weather, soil, disease patterns and mortality trends, drink and its effects, diet, diversions, medical techniques, meteors, comets, rainfall, frosts, heat, and a long list of other factors.[84] What had been conceived as a means to identify the epidemiological effects of a few factors – heat, cold, moisture, dryness, and emanations – threatened in Short's hands to become a boundless search for associations between the human organism and its environment. There was hardly anything that Short would exclude.

For himself, however, Short had in mind research into only a few of these associations. Inspired by Graunt and the political arithmeticians more than by Sydenham, and concerned with disease in any form rather than only with epidemics, he would focus on a few variables, and especially on matters about which the disease and mortality registers he could consult would provide information.[85] He would, for instance, compare the ratio of christenings to burials in a given locale over time in order to deduce whether the salubrity of the place was changing. He thus outlined a programme of research similar to that followed in much present-day social and economic historiography: collect population data and compare them with information on prices, crops, weather, and season to discover links.[86] Short expected to find an explanation for the prevailing diseases and demographic ratios of a locale in its terrain and climate. Regions with the highest ratios of christenings to burials he found to be dry, open, rocky, and mountainous areas, and those with the lowest ratios he found 'especially on stiff Clay, rotten Earth, or near a Level with the Sea, great Rivers, Marshes, Lakes, or putrid Standing Waters'.[87] He thus reaffirmed what most environmentalists since Sydenham had taken to be the single most helpful observation in Hippocrates: it is chiefly the capacity or tendency of the air to absorb and hold moisture and other substances that determines its salubrity or insalubrity.

In the final analysis, however, Short departed from Arbuthnot's procedural recommendations in a way that hindered and obfuscated the pursuit of evidence about the environmental hypothesis. In the first place, he specified many things worthy of notice but he did not suggest how they might all be classified, or how information about them might be organised. And because he adopted, as technique of characterisation, loosely descriptive words and phrases whose relationship to one another remained unspecified and whose manner of representing phenomena or the characteristics of phenomena varied from one usage to another, Short would shift environmentalism away from the quantitative methodology recommended by Arbuthnot and back toward the qualitative language of Hippocrates and Sydenham. Of course the phenomena upon which Short chose to focus attention (soil type, altitude, and terrain) were not as open to quantitative characterisation as the factors identified by Arbuthnot. But the very choice of phenomena that could not be reduced to quantitative expression moved Short away from rather than toward a test of the hypothesis that epidemic disease is a function of environmental conditions. Moreover, Short turned to extracting moral rather than medical conclusions from his observations, specifically to a denunciation of 'Whoredom, Adultery, Drunkenness and Idleness' and other social ills.[88] In his last contribution to the field, *A Comparative History of the Increase and Decrease of Mankind in England and Several Countries Abroad*, Short concluded that London's high mortality rate could be explained by moral perversion rather than by environmental factors.[89]

Many things needed to be changed if mortality were everywhere to be reduced to its lowest possible rate, and if population growth were to be encouraged in keeping with the biblical injunction that mankind should increase. Short would refine behaviour, but he would also call attention to the medical benefits of London's wide and regularly washed streets,[90] and single out those features of terrain unsuitable for habitation. He would also divide the commons among the poor, prohibit large national debts (especially when held by foreigners), end grain exports, secure property and liberty, maintain a powerful army, and rigidly execute the laws.[91] In a word, Short's list of responses was as long as his list of things to be observed. In mentioning everything, he muddled the issue of testing or specifying the environmentalist hypothesis, and he also muddled the issue of deciding what most efficaciously to do.

With this step away from clarity Short brought to a close what may be styled the British phase of the medicine of the environment. After 1750 many British physicians would add research contributions, and reassert some features of the argument for intruding upon the environment's influence over disease. But the centre of investigation shifted to the continent. There, Arbuthnot's recommendations about the variables to be considered and the methodology to be used in considering them would lead to a more coherent search for the associations between environment and disease, and to a more coherent campaign to act.

CONCLUSION

Between 1660 and 1750 British physicians distinguished a question worthy of investigation in the search for a more efficacious medicine, and proposed the sources of information and the methodologies to be explored in seeking an answer. In the process they drew upon a classical medical tradition which blended with rather than departing from existing hypotheses about the origins of epidemic disease. The environmental ideas taken from Hippocrates were joined with new methodologies and tools. The most notable of these were mathematical expectation, which provided a means to detect historical patterns and project those into the future; demographic statistics – the counting and measuring urged by John Graunt and William Petty – who also pioneered in interpreting such population data as were already available; and meteorological data, open to collection because of the recent development of new instruments and open to interpretation in association with disease and mortality by means of mathematical expectation. Because new information and methodologies were added to the consideration of an old idea, the combination might have produced a rethinking of the old idea that separated it more clearly and more usefully from its blending with existing notions about the origins of epidemic disease. But in the British phase that did not happen. The validity of the theory was assumed, even while data additions and tests were proposed.

However, British environmentalism produced one significant deviation from the Hippocratic tradition. Whereas *Airs, Waters and Places* failed to identify any correctives to the environmental complex as encountered except – by implication and only by implication – the physician's treatment of a patient affected by it, British environmentalism distinguished an array of responses for correction and avoidance. Courses of medical treatment were made more explicit but, more important, the environmental constitution ceased to be considered fatalistically. It came to be seen as a factor susceptible to control and manipulation. Three responses seemed especially promising: drainage, the elimination of standing waters identified with heavy morbidity and mortality; lavation, the cleansing of streets and public areas; and ventilation, the creation of air circulation in closed quarters. Each of these will receive separate treatment, as will also a fourth measure added by continental environmentalists.

2 Medical Geography and Medical Climatology

> The public health is the vigour, the strength, the wealth, and the prosperity of a state.
>
> Menuret de Chambaud

> Preventive medicine, which seeks to destroy the causes of disease or to prevent it, is without doubt the most useful medicine.[1]
>
> Audin-Rouvière

A medicine of the environment emerged on the European continent between 1690 and 1710.[2] The leading figures in this formative stage, Bernardino Ramazzini, Giovanni Lancisi, and Friedrich Hoffmann, drew on what they knew of British work in medicine, political arithmetic, and the natural sciences in general, and added distinctive elements of their own. This chapter will describe these assimilations and additions, and examine a loop in the road we are following. Whereas in the first phase of environmentalism – the phase of Sydenham and Arbuthnot – the identification of forces and factors deemed relevant to the environment–disease association expanded, ultimately, to the confusion of Short's unbounded list, continental interest focused on either a medicine of places or a medicine of climates. By specialising, this interest forced the medical effort into a more thorough exploration of central propositions, and away from a mere listing of all the potentially relevant variables. Continental environmentalism sought to record specific symptoms and characteristics of the milieu and to schematise the signs and signals of the milieu about disease.

Specialisation reaffirmed the environmental hypothesis, not because it failed to produce evidence flatly in conflict with the association, but because it produced a body of data too large to be absorbed. It also seemed to confirm the efficacy of the medicine of avoidance, and the specific steps of avoidance and environmental manipulation recommended by Sydenham, Boyle, Arbuthnot, Short and the other British environmentalists. In this phase, therefore, the medicine of the environment (endorsed by some of the great medical authorities of the day) was broadcast until it became general in Europe. Before the middle of the eighteenth century the medical literature of lands from the Mediterranean to Scandinavia, and from central Europe to the Atlantic coast and beyond, to North America, was rich in its enthusiasm for this means of explaining epidemic disease. Let us follow the development of this enthusiasm.

RAMAZZINI AND HOFFMANN

The premier exponent of environmentalism in the decades surrounding the turn from the seventeenth to the eighteenth century was the Modena physician Bernardino Ramazzini. Working within a rich Italian tradition of concern with the effects of external influences upon health, character, and temperament, Ramazzini examined the diseases and other characteristics of people performing certain occupations, and compiled a barometric diary and a series of disease and weather investigations of Modena. The study of occupational disease, *De morbis artificum*, Ramazzini's best known work, brought to a culmination a long list of Italian writing dating back to the fifteenth century.[3] His investigations of the epidemic constitution of Modena helped inaugurate a fresh variation on the old theme.

British environmentalists were familiar with parts of this work, and in Ramazzini's later study of occupational disease it is evident that the physician of Modena knew Boyle's writings. But it is not clear how much Ramazzini was influenced by British work before 1690, when his first study of the epidemic constitution appeared. On a visit to Modena in 1689, Wilhelm Leibniz discussed barometric and hydrostatic problems with Ramazzini.[4] Halley's recent work may also have entered this discussion. Perhaps Leibniz mentioned his expansion on Petty's political arithmetic, specifically his unsuccessful promotion of a centre for gathering vital statistics that would include a medical council.

For this project Leibniz formulated fifty-six questions dealing, in part, with the relationship between disease and environment. Whether or not Leibniz and Ramazzini discussed all these matters, Leibniz' attachment to the ideas of Sydenham and Petty helps account for the more or less simultaneous development of interest in the meteorological approach identified by Sydenham and followed by Locke, Boyle, and others. Leibniz, who made some small contributions of his own to environmental pathology, played a leading role in an international network of scientific discourse through which precisely such ideas were disseminated.

Studying conditions in the vicinity of Modena in the spring and summer of 1690, Ramazzini attributed a malaria epidemic that began in April to the influence of environmental forces – floods, stagnant waters, acid particles in the air, and prevailing north winds. At the year's end, as dry weather set in, the epidemic ended. To circulate his account and analysis of these events, Ramazzini wrote the first of three similar studies, *Constitutio epidemica ruralis*. In 1691 he reported on that year's conditions, and in 1695 on the epidemic constitution of 1692–4. The epidemics of 1690 and 1691 looked like straightforward products of environmental conditions. But the causal nexus of 1692–4 was more complicated, and Ramazzini's meteorological journals, kept simultaneously, did not clarify the causal framework. Ramazzini thus recommended the compilation of additional epidemic histories which would clarify how atmospheric conditions produce epidemics.[5]

But Ramazzini was soon distracted. Not until 1709, after a severe cold experienced in much of Europe during December 1708–March 1709, did he return to the study of environmental epidemiology. This was the same weather to which Lancisi in Rome attributed a 'rheumatic epidemic'. Ramazzini, turning again to Hippocrates, predicted a summer wave of acute fever, and spent the remainder of the term lecturing on that malady.[6]

The same extraordinary cold, which has drawn the attention of historians interested in the great harvest failure of 1709, puzzled Friedrich Hoffmann, then serving as court physician to Frederick I in Berlin. Hoffmann's interest in Hippocratic ideas about the environment may have been sparked during travels in France, the Netherlands, and England in 1684–5, during which he met and became friendly with Robert Boyle.[7] After being appointed professor of medicine at Halle, Hoffmann adopted Ramazzini's (and Sydenham's) tack in describing the influence of meteorological conditions on an epidemic in Halle in 1700.[8] Five years later he served as praeses (with J. B. Hoffstadt as respondent) for *Dissertatio de morbis certes regionibus et populis propriis*, which attempted to sketch a geography of disease through research in travel literature.[9] These two books, the study of Halle's 1700 epidemic constitution and Hoffstadt's dissertation, may also have been influenced by Ramazzini, who had sent Leibniz a copy of his 1691 description of Modena's epidemic constitution. Leibniz was much impressed with this work, and recommended it as a model for German physicians to emulate.[10]

Despite his meteorological investigations, Hoffmann's ideas about the pathogenic environment developed along a different path from that followed in Britain. Adhering more strictly to Hippocratic tradition, Hoffmann sought to identify the prevailing diseases of certain locales rather than to clarify understanding of the causal mechanism behind those associations. This was medical geography, not itself a new field, for German and Italian physicians had previously written about the prevailing diseases of certain locales. Indeed ten years earlier, in 1695, Lucas Schroeck, editor of the *Ephemerides* of the Vienna Academy of Science, had begun publication of a collection of studies by German physicians following Ramazzini's model.[11] But Hoffman opened this kind of inquiry to influence from the more ambitious programme of British environmentalism. If, in this way, Hoffmann's interests were narrower, they were also broader. The 1705 thesis which he directed sought to describe, albeit in only thirty-two pages, not the endemic diseases of a single place but those of Europe and the world. Hoffmann foresaw a universal medical geography, although he and Hoffstadt lacked the evidence to create such a comprehensive treatise.

Both the things that he did and the things that he did not do differentiated German medical geography from other varieties of environmentalism. Although in other writing Hoffmann professed to follow 'a simple clear mathematical method',[12] his conception of mathematics dealt with logic rather than arithmetic. Medical statistics and political arithmetic did not enter his sense of relevant procedures, nor did the gathering of quantitative characterisations of weather and climate. Moreover, although Hoffmann appealed to the Hippocratic advice to know nature, he considered the operation of environmental factors wholly within the conventional understanding of the non-naturals, those six influences identified in classical writing as necessary to health. In his writings humoural pathology gave way to a mechanical image of the body, and to corpuscular theory, but disease was still perceived as caused by the action of air or diet or another remote force on the balance of particles within the bodily fluids.[13] Hoffmann thus accepted atmospheric and general environmental conditions as a datum. He remained preoccupied with curative rather than preventive medicine.[14]

In the final analysis Hoffmann's environmentalism is seen to have been weaker than his attachment to other elements of the Hippocratic and Galenic traditions. In this sense he anticipated the views of the great Boerhaave who, like Hoffmann, shared many of the assumptions of environmentalism. But in Boerhaave's system these issues were even more muted than they were in Hoffmann's system.[15] Boerhaave's chief contribution to environmentalism was to be tolerant of it, and his tolerance helped give the theory credibility among the international cadre of physicians that he trained. Later environmentalists cited Boerhaave as belonging to the same tradition as themselves,[16] but in so doing they overlooked the central importance that Boerhaave attached to the course rather than the cause of disease.[17] Boerhaave regarded climate as one of the non-naturals, and therefore as an accessory rather than a proximate cause of disease. As a clinician, he was interested most in proximate causes. To the environmentalists, however, Boerhaave's proximate causes looked suspiciously like the disease itself. The dominance within European medicine in the 1720s and 1730s of the Leyden medical faculty did more to stunt than to assist environmentalism. This is most clear in Edinburgh, where Boerhaave's influence was great. In 1733 Arbuthnot had pointed to the newly developing medical faculty at Edinburgh as an important contributor to environmentalism. But as the influence of Boerhaave's students there grew, environmentalist studies languished.

Certain forms of environmental pathology, especially medical geography, continued to be practised during this era of Boerhaave. But only after Boerhaave's death, in 1738, did environmentalism emerge once again as a central stream of medical inquiry, as it had been in the two decades after 1690. In the 1740s and 1750s environmentalist arguments became more common, and their authors, who customarily cited Ramazzini and Hoffmann, began also to refer to Sydenham and Arbuthnot.[18] From the British point of view, environmentalism had already been an international movement in 1733, when Arbuthnot discussed a broad array of work in the field. By the middle of the century, continental and British environmentalists alike saw themselves as participants in the same cosmopolitan movement that Arbuthnot, somewhat prematurely, had detected.[19]

THE MEDICINE OF PLACES

The representative form of environmentalist writing in the 1730s and 1740s resembles a chiefly qualitative version of the work of Thomas Short, except in that it sought typically to characterise the medical geography of one city or one locale rather than to compile data about any and all regions.[20] These books, articles, and tracts reflect a particular interest in medical geography, which is to say that they pushed meteorological factors into the background and brought geographical and topographical factors into the foreground. Medical geography flourished especially in Germany, although examples of it may be found in a much larger area stretching from Siberia to the colonies of North America.

Burggrave and Behrends

German medical geography possessed a special interest in hygiene and sanitation. Its practitioners claimed that the urban improvements adopted by sixteenth-century German cities on the model of Renaissance Italian cities had fallen into decay. They wished also to draw the increasingly important central governments of eighteenth-century Germany into a revived campaign for public hygiene and sanitation. Let us consider these characteristics of the medicine of places by investigating the writings of two physicians. Both men practised in Frankfurt am Main and wrote medical geographies. Johann Philipp Burggrave published his book, *De aere & locis urbis Francofurtanae ad Moenum commentatio*, in 1751. Johann Adolph Behrends published *Der Einwohner in Frankfurt am Mayn in Absicht auf seine Fruchtbarkeit,*

Mortalität und Gesundheit geschildert twenty years later. They have much in common with each other, and some things in common with fellow environmentalists concerned especially with climate rather than place. But we shall look into the fresh things they have to say.

Burggrave shared with Hippocrates the desire to instruct inexperienced physicians. And he wished to be more specific, to do more than pass along the standard set of aphorisms, such as Hoffmann's 'change in air is often a remedy for severe diseases'.[21] Behrends, in contrast, wanted to instruct the lay public lacking access to physicians.

Among German environmentalists it was Burggrave who introduced medical statistics, considering population size and certain vital statistics in association with topography and other environmental features.[22] He thus drew into the service of medical geography the statistical investigations of Johann Peter Süssmilch, the Lutheran cleric who in 1741 had published an extended study of population experience which he supposed to reveal the demographic manifestations of divine design.[23] Using Süssmilch's reports, Burggrave could infer that Frankfurt was healthier than other German cities because it appeared to have a lower rate of mortality, and also because (adjusted for migration) the number of births considerably exceeded that of deaths. Like other eighteenth-century students of population, Burggrave could not find satisfactory information about migration. His adjustment was thus more intuitive than empirical. Once again, we see that the statistical data of medical geography were not always reliable. Burggrave's aggregates, which he inferred from Frankfurt records, may be seriously in error. Nevertheless the objective here is not to point out faulty data and statistical assumptions but to consider the inferences drawn by physicians from those data and assumptions. Burggrave detected certain peculiarities of the population and region of Frankfurt, and identified some disorders as common (for example, intermittent fevers) and others as uncommon (for example, smallpox). For the travelling physician of Hippocratic tradition (Burggrave moved to Frankfurt from Lombardy), this was useful work as an aid to diagnosis.

Although in some respects the Frankfurt of 1770, when Behrends wrote, seemed still to be more favoured than other German cities, Behrends was concerned not to blow the trumpet of civic pride but to find explanations for Frankfurt's deficiencies. The measure of those he found in a statistical survey that compared Frankfurt with Süssmilch's data, updated and expanded in a 1761–2 edition of *Die göttliche Ordnung*, on the experience of large-group averages in various population densities. In Frankfurt, for instance, marriage, christening, and burial registers were available for the period since 1670. They showed a recent decline in the ratio of marriages to christenings, and perhaps a slight fall in the absolute number of marriages. (Süssmilch had adopted the often misleading practice of reporting demographic data in the form of such ratios, and had thus overlooked the importance of differences in age structure.) Worse, the ratios indicated a sharp increase in the number of burials in comparison to christenings, which seemed to suggest that, since the mid-1740s, living conditions in Frankfurt had deteriorated.[24] Looking elsewhere, Behrends found marriage–population ratios much lower in other cities than in Frankfurt where (during each of the previous forty-six years) an average of only one marriage had been celebrated for each 170 people. Christenings, too, occurred in Frankfurt in smaller proportion than elsewhere. It was, he concluded, a case of excessive luxury, of ostentation, and of uncommonly high prices for the necessities of life. These things made marriage unattractive, especially to lower income groups. The frugality of old needed restoring.

In contrast, Frankfurt seemed to enjoy a lower mortality rate than other cities.[25] Even in the epidemic-ridden years of French occupation during the Seven Years' War (1756–63), the mortality–population ratio had risen merely to London's level. High fecundity offered another indication of the favoured situation of the city and its people. As against some temporary social and economic circumstances tending to depress population, Behrends found a variety of natural and man-made conditions tending to promote health and longevity. These he sought to identify so that less favoured cities might mimic Frankfurt.

Whereas Burggrave had set out to examine sickness and its cure, in the standard formulation of medicine and the initial formulation of the medicine of the environment, Behrends turned the quest upside down. Having established the greater healthiness of the city, he would examine the health-conducive features of its milieu. This was the rationale behind his lengthy description of terrain, climate and weather, and other aspects of the habitat.[26] Some phenomena, like the direction and force of the wind, defy manipulation, and in general climate and weather seemed less vital because they offered fewer opportunities for modification. Even harmful climatic forces might, however, be countered by avoidance or modification, for instance via dress or by laying out streets in a certain way (to take advantage of the wind direction).[27] The literature of historical epidemiology and of travellers attuned to medical issues left no doubt about the optimal city plan: widely spaced houses along broad streets regularly cleansed of rubbish and laid out so as to give the prevailing wind a free path.[28] Old cities, which could not afford such modifications, might still do some things beneficial to public health. Behrends recommended the elimination of moats, ditches, and other sites collecting standing water whose unhealthy emanations the breeze carried to neighbouring areas. In Frankfurt illnesses in the orphanage especially could be reduced by filling in sites in its vicinity where stagnant waters collected. Burggrave had detected the prevalence of intermittent fevers (presumably malaria) in and around Frankfurt. Behrends proposed what to do to avoid this disorder.

Behrends' views on public health improvements call to mind the long-standing concern of urban officials in Germany with the cleanliness of the city. To existing justifications for measures long recommended but not systematically pursued, Behrends added the arguments of environmental pathology. When he attacked the accumulation of animal refuse at tanneries and slaughterhouses, or pollution from textile washing and bleaching industries, and when he suggested that burials within Frankfurt cease, he did so on grounds of a specific theory about how refuse, pollution, and corpses were disease-conducive and with a specific promise about the benefits that would follow from improvements: the number and severity of epidemics would diminish.

Whereas Arbuthnot, of all the environmentalists, had sought most avidly to penetrate the properties and qualities of the air, Behrends, who had read Arbuthnot, focused also on water. In a fashion analogous to the capacity of the air to cleanse through ventilation, water acted through lavation – the cleansing wash. It is also, as a drink, an important contributor to good health or its absence. Behrends believed the effects of water to vary according to the weight and content of water in a given locale. Chemical and physical experiments revealed a variety of properties in Frankfurt's water, and suggested distinctions as to healthiness among parts of the city using water from different sources. And the choice of drinking water, more so than of air, is open.[29] To the inhabitants of Frankfurt Behrends recommended a number of improvements to reduce mortality and enhance healthiness. Where Burggrave had sought to teach physicians how better to treat the common ailments of the city, Behrends wished to teach the city's inhabitants how not to get sick in large numbers in the first place. The medicine of places had become statistical in its search for evidence, and had shifted emphasis away from reactive treatment and toward avoidance and prevention.

Finke and Frank

Between 1751, when Burggrave published, and the end of the eighteenth century, medical geographies were compiled for Erfurt (twice), Strasbourg, Stendal, Königsberg (now Kaliningrad), Berlin, Hamburg (by the French refugee Menuret de Chambaud), and a number of other towns and regions.[30] To Leonhard Ludwig Finke, reflecting on such matters in 1780, after four years of a bilious fever epidemic in Tecklenburg, where he was medical officer, these were medical topographies rather than medical geographies. They dealt with delimited regions. What was wanting was a general medical and practical geography, which Finke set out to prepare and published in 1792–5. With a limited array of sources at his disposal, and relying heavily on travel literature, Finke sought nevertheless to bring the goal of Hoffmann and Hoffstadt to fruition by dealing with the entire world. Introducing the third volume, he attempted also to formulate some general principles for preparing medical topographies – advising, for instance, that his often uncritical use of travel literature to devise descriptive commentaries be superseded by more heavily quantitative measurements.[31] This was, Finke acknowledged, a preliminary synthesis, a preliminary map of world disease. Too much of the globe awaited investigation after the manner of the medical topographers to allow more than tentative conclusions. But it was time to lend a common method to the investigation, to establish a syllabus of questions, to prepare a manual for the topographer.

Of Finke's work we should notice that he set out to sketch a universal medical topography before he had more than the most general of notions about which mechanisms might be at work in the disease-conducive features of human habitats. Like his predecessors, therefore, Finke deferred the matter of carefully scrutinising the assumptions upon which his manual was based. Both features – his scheme of doing medical topographies and his deferral of a critical scrutiny of environmentalist assumptions – influenced nineteenth-century German epidemiology. The medical topography remained a common form of medical investigation until nearly the end of the nineteenth century; throughout, the topographers followed Finke in reporting their observations rather than using them to test the theory behind their activities.

Finke wished especially to organise the sustained inquiries that would reveal all the elements and all the subtleties of the environment–disease association on a global front. But he interested himself also in discovering the correctable defects of the environment, and to that end assisted Johann Peter Frank in the opening stages of Frank's effort to compile a manual on how to prevent disease and promote health.[32] Frank, a public health physician and director of Viennese hospitals, was not a medical geographer or topographer. He was instead an administrator of environmentalism whose sustained barrage of suggestions for public health improvements, and for a medical police, drew upon both the traditional German concern with hygiene and sanitation and upon many of the specific proposals of the medical topographers. Frank thus integrated the suggestion that tax incentives be used to spur the drainage of swamps and stagnant waters with his own notions about state regulation of medical training and licensing.[33] Whereas German medical geography had, up to the end of the eighteenth century, developed chiefly under private initiative, Frank foresaw a broad and paternalistic involvement of government in this and all other fields of policy making that might contribute to the ultimate goal of increasing the wealth and population of the state. In this Frank's work is distinctly unoriginal in its recommendations about public health improvements and in the general quest for more numerous and more prosperous populations. It is original in the idea of shifting responsibility for the endeavour to the state. Frank, a servant of Austria's enlightened despots (Joseph II and Leopold II), shared their views on the efficacy of state intervention.

Dispersal of the Medicine of Places

Under the leadership of German physicians, the medicine of places worked out in the eighteenth century a methodology for gathering data about the environment–disease characteristics of each locale, and iterated a lengthening list of measures that might disrupt this association. Not only German physicians interested themselves especially in the relationship between the topographical or geographical features of a region and its endemic and epidemic diseases. In North America William Currie sought in 1792 to provide a general medical topography of the continent, reporting what he had learned from physicians throughout the United States.[34] Currie might have drawn more extensively than he did on a rich tradition of research on circumscribed regions. He might, for example, have read the works of John Lining and Lionel Chalmers on Charleston, South Carolina. In a letter to the *Philosophical Transactions* published in 1753, Lining reported his research into rainfall at Charleston during 1738–52 as part of an effort to discover 'the changes made in a climate, by clearing the land of its woods'.[35] Chalmers, working a generation later, sketched the weather of South Carolina, 'and from thence endeavour[ed] to account, for the various diseases to which the inhabitants of that country are liable, in consequence of the changes which their constitutions undergo in the several seasons of the year'.[36] There was in America no specific tradition of a medicine of climates or of places, but rather a generalised search into a newly settled environment. To Europeans North America was especially interesting for what it revealed about how an initially hostile environment might be made friendly. Such questions interested Currie, who wished in *An Historical Account of the Climates and Diseases of the United States* to provide the first medical geography of North America, and to show how the circumstances of a place might be altered.[37]

For tropical areas inhabited by Europeans and for the long shipboard life of voyages to the West and East Indies, James Lind furnished one of a number of environmentalist studies.[38] Lind's theme was to urge Europeans to leave unhealthy climates and sites during their sickly seasons, removing themselves to 'dry, elevated, and well ventilated spots'.[39] More generally this literature, which overlapped with the medicine of climates, sought to deal with the problem of high mortality among Europeans, especially new arrivals, in these hostile settings. In the process it produced detailed examinations of the medical conditions peculiar to life on board ship and in hot climates, and some variations on suggestions by European environmentalists for modifying the habitat. These are a topic for later consideration. For the moment, the goal is to complete a survey of enough of this literature to reveal its universality in Europe and the European world.

In the Dutch Netherlands the Haarlem Academy of Science posed several competitions around environmentalist questions. One of them – What are the common diseases that result from the natural situation of the country? – was answered in 1778 by Iman Jacob van den Bosch. Although he could cite few Dutch predecessors in the field,[40] Van den Bosch set out at once to compile a medical geography of the Netherlands rather than a topography of a single region. The tradition of Hippocrates and Hoffmann,[41] in which he saw himself as working, inspired confidence in the validity of a general view of the diseases of the land. After the fashion of the demographer Süssmilch, Van den Bosch sought information from medical authorities throughout the Republic.[42] Their answers revealed a number of geographical alterations – such as the gradual sinking of the polders – that seemed to have pathological implications. Van den Bosch therefore recommended an array of improvements (among them new hydraulic engineering projects) that would meliorate the healthiness of sites adjacent to or near water, a situation all too common in the Netherlands.[43]

In Spain Miguel Marcelino Boix y Moliner introduced his colleagues to the revised interpretation of Hippocrates, and to the work of Sydenham and Boyle, in 1716.[44] During the century thereafter a number of physicians followed this lead, and in 1791 François Thiéry used their work to compile a collection of medical topographies.[45] Environmentalist studies with a topographical and geographical orientation may be found also in Sweden,[46] Poland,[47] Ireland, the Czech lands, Siberia, Minorca, Italy, France, and elsewhere. Other types of literature often furnished the occasion for environmentalist observations. Travel accounts continued to include epidemiological commentary in the tradition of Sloane's reports on Jamaica. One of the most important eighteenth-century works of this type is Alexander Russell's *Natural History of Aleppo*.[48] A physician, Russell could report with particular confidence on the diseases of the region, especially on the interesting cases of plague and a *mal d'Aleppo*, and thereby furnish other environmentalists with data they took to bolster their own interpretations and to give those interpretations still broader geographical validity.[49] Eighteenth-century demographic research also incorporated elements of environmental pathology. William Black's several works in medical statistics, which were published during the 1780s, contributed to the medical geography of Britain, and Jean-Baptiste Moheau's important work on French demography considered environmental issues.[50]

The medicine of places broadcast the idea that site has a special impact upon health and disease, and that sites may be modified to be made less disease-conducive. There are many books and articles in this literature; only a few of them have been mentioned. They will repay the historian of a region or locale by providing detailed information about the eighteenth-century setting, about which we know so little because subsequent generations have built on to and over the earlier sites. These sources therefore provide verbal pictures to complement the town views, so typical an expression of early modern civic pride. And they will often tell a great deal more than can be seen in images of buildings, for they reveal something about the people who lived in these buildings and the physicians who tended to their health. But the medical topographies and geographies are also too rich. They tell us more about the features of individual locales than we can assimilate, not so much because we lack the means to sort so much data as because we lack the means to detect equivalences within the individual approaches of eighteenth-century physicians. I have not attempted either to sort these vast data, or to convey fully the tedium of detail in so many books and articles dealing with variations large and small on the same theme. Later I shall pose some questions about the means of avoidance and prevention common to these sources. For the moment, let us leave them and turn our attention to the climatological counterpart of the medicine of places – the medicine of climates.

THE MEDICINE OF CLIMATES

If the medicine of places was above all a specialisation of German environmentalists, the medicine of climates finds its most developed expression in the work of French physicians. Like the German expression of environmentalism, French interest in the association between the habitat and epidemic disease overlapped with other themes. But it stressed the influence of climatic factors on health. Whereas the German topographers focused on the natural history of the locale, the French made climate and weather the primary features to be described and quantified. The French also wrote what they called medical topographies, but in those they usually treated site succinctly and climate at length.[51]

Toward the middle of the eighteenth century interest in environmentalist issues quickened in France and elsewhere. The first signs of this in France are found in the 1740's in Mairan's call to the Académie royale des sciences for a massive collection of data to improve medical science, in Paul-Joseph Malouin's 'Histoire des maladies épidémiques de 1746', and in Antoine Deparcieux the elder's appeal for a national survey of infant life expectancy that would determine the healthiest regions within France.[52] The response was abundant.

Let us investigate a representative of French research, someone who helped fashion the goal of French inquiry into the environment–disease association, who influenced later work in a major way.[53] Jean Razoux, a Montpellier-trained physician practicing at the Nîmes hôtel-dieu, compiled daily tables of clinical and weather phenomena from 1 June 1757 until 1761 and published those findings in *Tables nosologiques & météorologiques*.[54] Razoux' technique was that of the clinician who expects numerous observations to reveal interrelations among the disorders encountered, and to distinguish effective treatments. To this conventional expectation he added the idea of an expanded realm of observations (Razoux appears to have been unaware of British predecessors).[55] His goal was not only 'to make many observations at the bed of the patient, and to reason little' but also to examine nature, terrain, climate, weather, the character and manners of the citizens, diet, water and other potables, the illnesses of the seasons: all that once gathered will yield 'a practical system of medicine founded on experience of the most certain and authentic kind'.[56] In the design of his scheme Razoux consulted the great continental physicians of the day, Sauvages, Van Swieten, Tronchin, Allioni, La Condamine, and others. In extending his approval of the plan, Sauvages wrote that if anything were to improve medicine it would be 'a similar scheme carried out over fifty years by some thirty physicians who are equally precise'.[57]

In Nîmes Razoux found both a garrison of the royal army and an institution, the hôtel-dieu, serving without differentiation the sick, the disabled, and the destitute. The hôtel-dieu specialised, however, in treating soldiers and the citizens of the municipality. As physician there Razoux was well placed to amass quickly a large number and wide variety of case histories.[58] In the style that became standard among French environmentalist studies, Razoux opened his book with a description of Nîmes and its setting, the characteristics of its inhabitants, and the common diseases of the area. But he turned quickly (and devoted most space) to climate and weather observations. His Nîmes meteorological readings give barometic pressure, temperature, wind direction, and general comments on the weather; the separate nosological tables give type of illness, observations thereon, symptoms, treatments, and statistics on admittances, the number cured, convalescent, and dead within the month. In June 1757, for example, of 167 male patients, 116 were discharged as cured, 5 died, and 46 remained to convalesce; among 35 females (with a separate hall) 27 were cured, 5 died, and 3 remained to convalesce.[59] Razoux' nosological record omits certain months, but for twenty-seven of fifty-five months for which totals are given, the Nîmes hôtel-dieu accepted 5 092 patients. Of those 4 663 (92 per cent) were released as cured, 406 (8 per cent) died, and 23 (less than 1 per cent) are unaccounted for.[60]

Could the Nîmes hôtel-dieu have been such a benign, indeed healthy, place? Will these records suggest anything about the efficacy of hospital care in the eighteenth century, and will they tend to contradict the customarily bleak picture of hospitals? Razoux was, of course, an interested observer who might have wanted to show this institution in the best light. Its patients were selected, but the grounds for this selection are not fully explained. Among townspeople, as Razoux claims, all segments of the male population used the hôtel-dieu. Since for most age groups (perhaps for all but very advanced ages), male mortality exceeded female, the preference for male patients should have increased the loss rate. But the hôtel-dieu's patients were disproportionately soldiers rather than civilians. In some circumstances eighteenth-century soldiers are known to have had much higher morbidity and mortality rates than civilians,[61] so that the remarkable success of the Nîmes hôtel-dieu in curing patients might be accounted for by nothing more mysterious than malingering within the garrison. This is, of course, merely speculation. But it does warn us against generalising from Peuchet's reports about the very hazardous Paris health institutions of the early nineteenth century.[62] Razoux' work is a small contribution to two problems: reconstructing rates of morbidity within the general population of the old regime, and establishing the incidence of mortality within institutions designed to care for the sick as well as others.

Razoux compiled a staggering volume of information, aggregated and tabularised. It was, nevertheless, only the record of one institution over a few years. As Sauvages had foreseen, one should expect the law of large numbers to apply in medical climatology as in other variables of statistical investigation – the larger the quantity of data the smaller the margin of error. Sauvages would have preferred a large and bold venture – thirty physicians working for fifty years. But both the French public and royal officials held mixed views about the collection of vital statistics. State officials saw it as a valuable but costly exercise that might, moreover, lead to potentially dangerous findings. Was the population, and thus the potential military force, really as large as estimated without enumerative surveys? The public at large was generally unsympathetic to any inquiry of this sort, seeing it as a harbinger of increased taxation or as a violation of divine order that would provoke another visitation of the sort experienced by the Israelites after David's census.[63] Both reactions would reveal themselves in the *enquête* launched under the direction of Félix Vicq d'Azyr, a Parisian anatomist.

In 1776 the controller general of finances (Turgot) appointed a commission to investigate the causes of epidemic and epizootic diseases, and recommend means of control and prevention.[64] The immediate occasion for this step was the persistent livestock epizootic of 1770–6. Out of the commission emerged in 1778 the Société royale de médecine which, with funding from the treasury, set out to compile a medical climatology and topography of the entire kingdom. Using questionnaires and organising a general search for information from provincial and Parisian physicians, the *enquête* would collect data on epidemics and epizootics and the means of treatment applied to them. It would also 'investigate the connection that may exist between the succession of the seasons and epidemics; then establish a catalogue of geographical circumstances that will eventually help form a pathological cartography; finally find in what measure "epidemics seem sometimes to spare one group of citizens", or even entire nations'.[65]

Between 1776 and 1792 the *enquête* led to the collection of an unmanageably large body of information. From Normandy, for example, the physician Lépecq de La Clôture sent his 1 076 pages of 'observations sur les maladies et constitutions épidémiques', which the Society published, at the king's expense.[66] Some of the data gathered in the *enquête* were included in reports prepared each year by the meteorologist Père Louis Cotte for the Society's *Histoire*. Others were at least remarked upon in print. But the resources and statistical techniques at Vicq d'Azyr's disposal were not adequate even to aggregate and tabularise so much information, much less to search through it for the correlations the participants expected to find. Nevertheless it was not a sense of an excessive bulk of data that daunted French physicians at the end of the century so much as a continuing sense of the scope of information that needed to be collected and analysed. In 1799 J.-B. Demangeon added new issues to the list of relevant variables: dress, people's interests, physical and moral education.[67] Like Thomas Short half a century earlier, Demangeon saw no boundary around the influences that should be deemed relevant.

A PERIOD OF SCEPTICISM

To ask more questions was to call for more data about the environment–disease association. Implicitly, as we can see in retrospect, asking for more information indicated a feeling that the data which had been gathered had not fully revealed the associations those data had been expected to clarify. The medicine of the environment entered a mild crisis of confidence toward the end of the eighteenth century, but this was not a crisis of overtly recognised failures in the research plan. The environmentalists remained confident that more data would reveal and clarify. The things they worried about were instead comparatively technical issues which, as a group, seemed to indicate that unravelling the association between climate and disease or between site and disease would be still more complex than had been supposed.

One form of this crisis of confidence is to be found in misgivings about the reliability of the information which so much effort had been expended to gather. The Leyden-trained physician William Black, unhappy in 1780s with the still deficiently quantitative content of environmentalism, proposed to create 'the science of Medical Arithmetick and Universal Prognosticks'.[68] Black would explicitly apply the law of large numbers to medical statistics and quantify hitherto qualitative data in order to build a nosology incorporating statistical data about the incidence of disease and death with information on location and population density. But the only available body of information of this sort – the London bills of mortality – Black found so defective that he felt it necessary to undertake the prior step of improving the means of collecting mortality data.[69] In short, Black wanted, more than a century after Sydenham, to start afresh with data collection.

Another area of rising scepticism may be found in meteorology. The instruments and techniques devised especially in the seventeenth century had seemed to promise a fruitful arena for the collection of observations that would sooner or later reveal the laws of climate and weather, and the laws of climatological disease. But a long era of data collection had failed either to explain climate and weather or to ground firmly the matter of prediction. In a long and important preface to an Italian translation of Abraham de Moivre's study of probability, Roberto Gaeta and Gregorio Fontana maintained that meteorological observations had done nothing more than serve frivolous hypotheses.[70] This was also d'Alemberts's view. Not everyone wondered about the efficacy of gathering weather observations, for meteorological societies that did nothing else continued to exist, and leading thinkers of the age mimicked Locke in keeping weather diaries. But the first questions about the ultimate contribution of this effort to knowledge had been asked.

Toward the end of the eighteenth century theories about

climatic influence, identified especially with Montesquieu, came under sustained attack. Conventional wisdom may be seen in the work of William Falconer of Bath.[71] While he disagreed with specific inferences Montesquieu had drawn from experiments on the effects of cold,[72] Falconer accepted most of Montesquieu's more general assumptions. At one with *Esprit des lois*, and with d'Alembert's article in the *Encyclopédie*, he repeated such old notions as the claim that hot climates promote indolence and timidity so that a hundred Europeans can whip a thousand Indian soldiers.[73] But in medicine Falconer's analysis was, when it appeared in 1781, already an anachronism, for environmentalists were focusing not on invariable effects of climate but on the variable effects of weather. What is most interesting is that the attack on climatic determinism as a system did not itself prompt scepticism about environmentalism.[74]

To this doubt Italian environmentalism added the failure of expectations for a new device intended to measure the mephitic – noxious, pestilential or foul-smelling – qualities of the air. In Italy the tradition of Ramazzini's study of the epidemic constitution remained strong throughout the eighteenth-century. Carlo Ricca studied the constitution of Turin in the early 1720s, and Paolo Valcarenghi that of Cremona in the late 1730s. For Naples Michele Sarcone examined the diseases of the year 1764 in detail. Rome, Padua, Florence and other cities also drew environmentalist consideration, chiefly under the aim of compiling a record of epidemiological experience. By the 1780s much work was being done under the influence of the Société royale de médecine in Paris, which affirmed the objectives that already dominated Italian environmentalism.

Beyond these standard works, however, Italian scientists contributed a new instrument designed to measure the qualities of the air at any site and therefore to distinguish areas requiring a quarantine of site.[75] On the basis of Joseph Priestley's 1774 assertion that the purity of the air may be evaluated by the proportion of dephlogisticated air (or oxygen) in it, Marsilio Landriani and Felice Fontana (and Priestley himself) built instruments which they called eudiometers. In place of the retrospective and therefore tardy morbid barometer provided by mortality data, the eudiometer, it was hoped, would furnish an anticipatory means of identifying disease-prone sites. Environmentalist physicians thus set out to collect eudiometer readings, thereby to distinguish healthy from unhealthy areas and also to grade the degree of unhealthiness in mephitic regions.[76] Quickly enough, however, eudiometer readings were found to vary only slightly, and then not in a pattern analogous to mortality. Furthermore, the pneumatic chemistry of Priestley, like Behrends' researches into the sediment in water, failed to show how to link atmospheric gases with disease.[77] As a device of environmentalism, use of the eudiometer faded within a decade of its invention.

This failure of the eudiometer to solve the problem of distinguishing the precise elements that made an unhealthy site unhealthy seems to have bolstered doubt about whether the structure and mechanics of the environment–disease association would ever be understood. Nevertheless the failure of this device, and more generally the failure of pneumatic chemistry, to specify the mephitic properties of the air, also did not lead to scepticism about environmentalist presuppositions. It led instead to a search in still other directions to identify the pathogenic features of the environment.

CONCLUSION

In this chapter the investigation has centred on the medicine of places, the medicine of climates, the universality of the environmentalist assumption, and late eighteenth-century doubts. Acceptance of the environment–disease association spread across Europe and beyond, as it spread across Britain, because the citation of classical sources strengthened faith in this hypothesis. But in most countries there was also one, or a few, great practitioner-theorists who lent credibility to the theory: in Britain and for much of Europe that role was played by Sydenham and, to a lesser extent, by Arbuthnot; in Germany by Hoffmann; in Italy by Ramazzini and Lancisi; in France by Sauvages. Before the middle of the eighteenth century many physicians in many lands shared the notion that group diseases arise from environmental conditions.

If we reflect for a moment on the contents of the writings encountered in this and the preceding chapter, we will notice how often the environmentalists were (in their own terms) empiricists – reporting their observations – and how seldom they speculated openly about how they drew the conclusions they did. In the next two chapters we shall have a chance to inquire further into their processes of reasoning. For the moment, it is more important to notice how often the process of adding to basic Hippocratic theory (and specifying it) proceeded in a manner that seems to us indirect or even unwitting. Sydenham's introduction to his consideration of London's epidemic constitutions of 1661–75 for the most part reports observations. It is nevertheless full of assumptions, assumptions that became fundamental in environmentalist theory because of Sydenham's influence. This implicit theorising appears in eighteenth-century sources as well. Following it, environmentalists selected what to study and what evidence to gather, and inferred what treatments or steps of avoidance and prevention their observations seemed to warrant. Since so many physicians accepted the environmentalist hypothesis as theory without being provided with proofs of it, we may assume that this explanation of epidemic disease seemed plausible because it agreed with so many predispositions – to see nature as subject to human manipulation, to organise and render statistical knowledge about disease and the habitat, to acknowledge situational and climatic variations.

Another feature to notice now is the shift of emphasis away from Sydenham's preeminent concern – finding efficacious treatments – toward the primary concern of mature environmentalism, detecting the pestilential aspects of the environment in order that they might be modified or avoided. More and more eighteenth-century epidemiology was a medicine of the environment, rather than of diseases. More and more the epidemiologist's gaze focused on the things around the patient, rather than on the patient. In the long run therefore it was less Sydenham than Ramazzini who influenced the development of environmental pathology. Where Sydenham had been pessimistic about the physician's capacity to find the means to avoid or prevent disease, Ramazzini had distinguished specific and practical measures to be taken. He expressed this hopeful view in his treatise of occupational diseases. 'We must admit that the workers in certain arts and crafts sometimes derive from them grave injuries' and 'dangerous diseases'.[78] In return for the contributions these workers make to civilisation, we should take 'precautions for their safety, so that as far as possible they may work at their chosen calling without loss of health'. Ramazzini had rather few corrective steps to suggest, but he possessed a strong faith that useful measures might be discovered and adopted.

Continental physicians reaffirmed both the long British list of potential associations between the environment and disease, and the short British list of efficacious actions. They, too, recommended drainage, lavation, and ventilation. But they added another species of action, so far mentioned only once. In Frankfurt Behrends wanted burials to occur outside the city, thus to isolate the dead from the living. This was not a new idea, and we notice it here only in passing – more will be said later. The argument behind the case for a new location for interment was to save the living from the emanations of the dead. The four leading measures of environmentalism – drainage, lavation, ventilation, and interment – are now complete.

Many sources have been mentioned and cited. They do not speak, of course, for the physicians who did not publish, or who did not publish books or essays that I have read. But they do speak loudly. Even if unpublished practitioners were discovered in as yet unknown sources to have had other ideas, or to have lacked interest in a medicine of avoidance or prevention, it should be evident by now that a large and vocal group of physicians believed in the environment–disease association, and believed also that they knew something about how to disrupt it, and were learning more.

We conclude, therefore, with an irony. The mild crisis of confidence that can be detected in late-century environmentalist writing did not undermine confidence in the theory or the efficacy of inferences from the theory. There was, if anything, a crisis of overconfidence. Environmentalists tended to believe that the hypothesis had already been tested and found accurate, or that impending tests would resolve any small doubts remaining. It is this overconfidence and the optimism associated with it which provides a theme for later chapters. In those we shall move away from the building blocks of environmentalist theory toward the actions of avoidance and prevention that the environmentalists recommended. When in 1798 Menuret de Chambaud described public health as 'the vigour, the strength, the wealth, and the prosperity of a state', he did so not merely because he wished to interest public authorities in improving health in general, but also because he believed that the means of improvement were known.[79]

3 Epidemiological and Environmental Surveillance: Counting and Measuring Pathogenic Signs

> I have often thought that if such a [meteorological] Register. . . were kept in every County in *England*, and so constantly published, many things relating to the Air, Winds, Health, Fruitfulness, &c. might by a sagacious man be collected from them, and several Rules and Observations concerning the extent of Winds and Rains, &c. be in time established, to the great advantage of Mankind.[1]
>
> Locke

The medicine of the environment seemed to many eighteenth-century physicians to provide a way to anticipate epidemic disease, and thus to block or elude its effects. In surveying some leading and representative selections from environmentalist literature from Sydenham to the end of the eighteenth century, we have seen that this idea was shared across Europe and regions of the globe inhabited by Europeans. Let us now probe more deeply into the methodology of observing the environment, and read both the lines and between the lines of our sources seeking insight into the mathematics and the statistical procedures of this inquiry.

MATHEMATICS AND OBSERVATIONS

The idea of analysing medical phenomena recorded in the form of aggregations rather than in enumerations of individual cases emerged in an explicit form in the latter decades of the seventeenth century. It should be traced to the merchant Graunt and the physician Petty who framed the first analytical questions about disease and mortality statistics. Already in 1662, in the first edition of *Natural and Political Observations. . .made upon the Bills of Mortality*, Graunt accepted a major premise of environmental pathology: acute and epidemic diseases occur 'suddenly and vehemently, upon the like corruptions and alterations in the Air'. This was not, we have noticed, a new idea. What was new in Graunt's consideration, as in that of the group of Anglo-Irish physicians and physicists identified with Sydenham, was the proposed response. Graunt wished to rank the major causes of death appearing in the London bills of mortality, and to examine the economic and demographic implications of London's mortality history. For him the disease totals were 'a Standard of healthfulness of the *Air*' and food of Londoners, which suggests that he approached these registers in much the same spirit that had motivated their initiation and other efforts in the late medieval and early modern period to record mortality and its trend.[2] The bills, like the books of the dead in Renaissance Florence, furnished a morbid barometer (although that particular metaphor of course emerged after the invention of the barometer by Torricelli in 1643).

William Petty was a formulator of intriguing questions. Interested especially in population quantities and economic resources – which data he believed would show that late seventeenth-century England was not in decline – Petty turned to burial and christening records as sources. From them he drew certain inferences about population density, its distribution by age, and comparative rates in different locales (e.g., London and Dublin). But Petty was dissatisfied with the reliability of christening and burial registers, and preferred that censuses be taken as a way of replacing these 'Ingenious, but very preposterous' substitute means of estimating population and its dynamics. Among the questions he posed for the census, Petty would ask about age, sex, cause of death, the last in preference in terms of his twenty-four categories and three headings of disease.[3] Thinking specifically of how to improve the Dublin bills of mortality, Petty wished to specify categories that would be easy to recognise, thereby to clear up the vexing problem of great diversity in causes of death as listed by the notoriously unreliable searchers of deaths. It will be apparent that replacing a long and often imaginative with a short list of causes of death would not have eliminated errors, and might indeed have made them more difficult to detect. What should be noticed is that Petty's proposal reflects his assumption, as a physician, of the existence of diseases as separable and distinct entities.

Sydenham was not entirely clear on this point. Winslow interprets his discussion of epidemic constitutions as indicating a conviction that the nature of a disease might change with its milieu.[4] In other writings Sydenham left no doubt about the different character of different diseases. But he also believed that changes in the environmental constitution would influence prevailing diseases, for example in their intensity. Even if physicians sometimes speculated about the existence of a disease continuum, they nonetheless accepted Petty's idea that a predominant cause of death might be specified for each individual. Therefore cause of death data could be gathered and compared from parish to parish 'in Order to know how the different Situation, Soil, and Way of living in each Parish, doth dispose Men' to different diseases.[5]

A prominent figure in the primitive formulation of statistical questions, and especially in sketching out a territory of distinctly medical statistics, Petty identified the kind of mortality data necessary for the environmentalist. He thus proposed new uses for the London bills. They would continue to provide a morbid barometer, but it would not be sufficient merely to add all the cases of plague deaths in order to compare those totals from week to week, as was commonly done. Knowing the trend and relative severity of plague mortality remained a useful thing, for it could indicate the appropriate timing of such measures of avoidance as Petty's scheme to transport Londoners into the countryside. But more useful still would be the discovery of how diseases are influenced by the environment. Petty saw that that could be done only by compiling data about both mortality by cause and the environment, in order to compare the two series.

Terminology

The procedure that Petty proposed came to be called a search for correlations. In Petty's day the words 'correlation' and 'correlative' had several meanings, all of which seem to have been established by, or during, the sixteenth century. These two words meant, in the first place, things occurring in conjunction. Then, as today, the intensity of the conjunctural relationship was not clearly established. At one end of the spectrum these words were used to suggest a reciprocal relation, such that one thing necessarily implies another. At the other end the relation was looser: a correlation was one thing normally related to or occurring along with something else. But these words were used also to mean 'analogous', which opened for them yet another range of definition. In the sense of things analogous, things correlative could refer to similarity, susceptibility to comparison, or parallelism. Used in that sense, the words 'correlation' and 'correlative' could imply the argument from analogy, which was such a powerful force in philosophical discourse in the seventeenth century.

By avoiding any use of the word 'cause', the *Oxford English Dictionary* creates the impression that sixteenth- and seventeenth-century usage of correlation and correlative had not developed a point of confusion that surrounds twentieth-century usage. These words were not yet used to suggest a causal relationship between, or among, the phenomena at issue. As Petty used the concept, phenomena in correlation with one another seem to have been meant to be seen as things in frequent or invariable accompaniment. But his adoption of the word 'dispose' ('how the different Situation. . .doth dispose Men') suggests a degree of causality. In the Hippocratic tradition the non-naturals were deemed necessary (i.e., inescapable) causes of disease. But it was also believed that their operation might not provide a sufficient or comprehensive explanation of disease.

By bringing this sense of causality together with the prevailing sense of phenomena in accompaniment with one another, Petty contributed to the development toward modern confusion about these two words, which mean such very different things to a statistician than to a humanist concerned with qualitative issues. In the eighteenth century this confusion existed without recognition. Environmentalists used 'correlation' and 'correlative' to suggest some degree of causality between the phenomena of the environment and those of epidemic disease, and sometimes also from disease to the environment and back to disease.[6] Only later would attention fall on the possibility that even things in invariable accompaniment with one another do not necessarily have any causal relationship. Hume pointed out the danger of jumping to the inference that causation is involved whenever two phenomena regularly recur in the same sequence, but he also associated causation preeminently with the contiguity of events.[7]

None of this discussion is meant to suggest that eighteenth-century medical statisticians ran tests to infer the degree of correlation, as a present-day statistician might do. The correlation coefficient had not yet been invented. The eighteenth-century search, lacking even the technique of the chart, which emerged only at the end of the eighteenth century,[8] sought to discern correlative relationships by eyeing the data annals – series of quantitative and qualitative data presented in chronological order.

Petty took the meaning of the word 'correlation' further toward a suggestion that the relationship between data in correlation is causal. Yet none of the weaker shades of association suggested in previous usages was discarded. In the eighteenth century, therefore, the search for data to be correlated was undertaken under the conviction that it would reveal how the environment caused, provided the occasion for (or intersected with) disease. All these senses of the nature of the relationship may be found in the literature, sometimes in close sequence.[9] William Hillary thus explained in the preface to his medical topography of Barbados that he was looking for how 'diseases were either influenced, caused, or changed' by weather variations.[10]

In addition to this unrecognised source of confusion, the medical literature of the eighteenth century reveals a recognised point of confusion. In 1724 the English physician George Cheyne, famous as the author of a handbook on good health, *An Essay to Health and Long Life*, denounced 'refined Speculations of Metaphysicks, or Mathematicks'. He preferred, he said, his own 'Experience and Observation'.[11] It was a point of pride for the 'modern' scientist of Cheyne's day to reject metaphysical speculation, as Newton had rejected that procedure, and to assert the superior merit of observation. But what did Cheyne mean by denouncing 'Mathematicks'? The context is revealing. Cheyne did not have in mind the arithmetic procedures that Petty used and recommended. In this case it is clear from the context that he had in mind a synonym for speculative reasoning.

When Arbuthnot published his *Essay on the Usefulness of Mathematical Learning* in 1701 he wished to make another distinction. The mathematics he wanted to foster was the mathematics of physics, political arithmetic, and mathematical expectation, in which he was expert. And Arbuthnot wanted to discredit iatromathematics, which appeared often in the form of medicine combined with astrology. Among the fields that would benefit from his version of mathematics Arbuthnoth included medicine. For some time thereafter the word 'mathematics' continued to be used for this wide range of meanings, and to be denounced by some physicians. It would be going too far to suggest that medicine adopted arithmetic while rejecting mathematics-as-speculation. What this discussion does indicate is that the frequently encountered attack on mathematics was not an attack on the medical statistics of the environmentalists, but on something else altogether.[12]

Gathering Observations

The environmentalist's goal was to observe, and to transform a sporadic into a rich historical record of observations. The sources available toward the end of the seventeenth century revealed remarkably little about the historical form of those phenomena deemed significant. Like Buffon in the *Histoire naturelle*, the environmentalist sought the exact description of everything,[13] an unremarkable aim because it was common to so many streams of scientific inquiry in the eighteenth century. The medical statistician thus shared the natural and the human scientist's sense that the available data were inadequate, that the task of science was to observe and record. From a vast knowledge of detail Locke's 'sagacious man' would find generalisations. Both the medical statistician and the natural scientist wanted to have a comprehensive data set. Both had to accept a number of compromises – in part because they had to depend chiefly on their own enterprise to gather data, and in part because their capacity to imagine potential data sets was too rich.

Which phenomena should be counted and measured? Petty

proposed situation, soil, way of living, and cause of death. Boyle, Locke, and Wren would add some meteorological phenomena, and Sydenham would focus on epidemics (as well as the signs of the epidemic constitution, which he did not distinguish). In the long run environmental pathologists would concern themselves especially with the three territories already identified: climate and weather, site, and disease. They would therefore push into the background a long list of possibly influential factors.

In the short run (up to about 1750), the chief problem the environmentalist faced was to gather reliable data. Some numerative records of these phenomena were already available in the 1670s, but those were sporadic in time and place: mortality registers for London but no analogous readings of the environment; temperature records for Padua but nothing of other meteorological phenomena or of disease. In Germany cause of death data were not compiled and published until 1719, when Johannes Daniel Gohl provided some statistics on Berlin in the *Acta medicorum berolinensium*.[14] Until the middle of the eighteenth century the nearly exclusive task of environmentalism was simply to compile simultaneous data sets. In the second half of the century, data sets accumulated. But some were separate records of climate and weather, site, or cause of death – useless without simultaneous records. Others failed to find their way into print, either in aggregated form or in interpretations. And still others found their way into print but did not immediately reveal the more specific environment–disease associations expected of them.

In collecting data medical statisticians confronted a number of problems that they were ill prepared to solve. The want of standardised meteorological instruments (or even of instruments able to give invariable readings under identical conditions) has been mentioned. Gordon Manley, the historical meteorologist, is struck by 'the extraordinary imperfections of both instruments and methods' in temperature measurement before 1750, and especially before 1700.[15] The environmentalists counted on these instruments to provide precise readings of weather phenomena, but they could not avoid having to use unreliable thermometers, barometers, and hydrometers. Moreover, they placed these instruments indoors and out, and read them at different times of the day and seldom with complete regularity. They could not adapt their practice of medicine and other activities to the regimen of meteorology.

To discern changes in the trend of morbidity, the medical statistician required not only data on death by cause but also information about the overall population and its age and sex structure. These needs matched those of the eighteenth-century demographer, who urged central governments to become involved in census taking.[16] Municipal and central governments often professed support for the collection of these data, and with increasing frequency ordered the gathering of data of some use to the medicine of the environment. But their motives were political and economic more often than scientific or medical. Governments wanted such data in order to determine the numbers of taxpayers or of fencible men, and to determine whether measures adopted to augment population or prosperity had had any effect. Moreover there was considerably more enthusiasm in government circles for the word than for the deed. Time and again French authorities ordered their agents in the provinces (the intendants) to collect basic data about the population and resources of their intendancies, and time and again the reports received were incomplete. Moreover, the reports as received were seldom published or otherwise made available to either demographers or medical statisticians. Only Sweden adopted a regular census during the eighteenth century, and made public the findings of the census, conducted by clerics.

Of the data sets already available, and those produced during the late seventeenth and the eighteenth century, large and serious errors concerned the analyst. Among the merits of Graunt's pioneering work is its criticism of the London bills. But the defects Graunt detected were not quickly corrected. Age at death data were not sought until 1728, and then remained imperfect if only because the living did not always know the age of the deceased, or even their own age. Writing more than a century after Graunt, William Black levelled many of the same charges of inaccuracy that Graunt had. These same defects are evident in the mortality data gathered in other locales. The demographers, Moheau in France and Süssmilch in Germany, were able to extract from ecclesiastical and other records some information about aggregate mortality. But most of these records failed to specify a cause of death. Moreover, although the key issue of epidemiology was the morbidity–environment association, none of the records supplied much information about even the trend of morbidity, such less about illness from specific diseases. The epidemiologist had to build his own data set without significant help from public, ecclesiastical, or other sources.

Some problems with statistical data were detected but unresolved, and other problems remained undetected. Behrends noticed that migration would influence the calculation of mortality and nuptiality ratios, and attempted to adjust for migration. But no one had any very dependable information about migration, so the foundations for these adjustments were intuitive or speculative. We have already noticed an important undetected problem: the failure of the demographer or the medical statistician to see that age structures of populations may vary, so that different mortality–population ratios in two cities may not signal different age-specific rates of mortality.

But the greatest problem was the failure of the environmentalist to combine serial information about the environment with morbidity data, or reliable and sufficiently numerous mortality-by-cause statistics. Like the eighteenth-century demographer, the medical statistician set out to gather data before thinking through his needs. The cumulative effect of these several kinds of difficulties is to render the statistical data of the eighteenth century seriously flawed. Historical statisticians in demography and economics, who have worked with eighteenth-century published accounts, have usually decided that it is necessary to undertake fresh aggregations from raw data. There is no doubt that the estimates of population, mortality trend, sex ratio, and other phenomena considered by the old regime demographers are superior to those wild guesses and vague qualitative assessments that had preceded them. French demographers before the Revolution of 1789 estimated the population at levels within 15 per cent of the reconstructions of present-day historical demographers, whereas their seventeenth-century predecessors had guessed the population of France in their day at as little as 5 million and as many as 48 million.[17] But neither the demographic nor the medical statistician was accurate enough to satisfy present-day demands, or systematically inaccurate in the same way. Here, however, the objective is not to reconstruct the pattern of mortality or morbidity and environmental circumstances, but to investigate how the old regime statisticians set out to gather data and the ways in which they interpreted their findings.

In pursuit of the information directly relevant to the medicine of the environment, John Locke joined in 1692 his fellow physician Charles Goodall in distributing questionnaires. Locke's part was to send the questionnaires to his wide circle of acquaintances and correspondents abroad. Goodall was to put the data together to discern the correlations they revealed, but he did not complete his task.[18] The questionnaires asked about mortality records, atmospheric conditions and changes in disease patterns perceived to occur with the seasons or atmospheric conditions, Sydenham's reputation and other issues. Without intending to do so, Locke and Goodall established a pattern for subsequent investigations. Time and again considerable effort would be expended on gathering data under the assumption that compilation and interpretation would readily follow. In truth, however, the environmentalist erred in believing that the major hurdle in elaborating and specifying the theory lay with data collection. It lay instead with deciding which data to gather, and how to interpret the data that were gathered.

John Lining

A fine illustration of these points may be found in the inquiries of John Lining, who practised medicine in Charleston, South Carolina. Trained in Scotland, Lining is identified with his 1753 description of the 1732 and 1748 yellow fever epidemics in Charleston. His study of his own metabolism is said also to have contributed to the problem of measuring insensible perspiration, which was an accounting device introduced in the seventeenth century to balance inputs and outputs in measuring metabolic signs.[19] In March 1740 Lining began constructing a series of what he called 'meteoro-statical tables', in which he recorded both weather data and information about his own bodily functions, the latter after the fashion of earlier experiments by Santorio Santorio with human and Stephen Hales with plant life.[20]

Lining expected that he 'might experimentally discover the Influences of our different Seasons upon the Human Body' and thereby 'arrive at some certain knowledge of the Causes of our epidemic Diseases, which as regularly return at their stated Seasons, as a good Clock strikes Twelve when the Sun is in the

Meridian'.[21] Such research seemed particularly appropriate for Charleston because the sharp changes of weather there would accentuate relationships that might otherwise go unnoticed. Lining accepted without reservation the notion that 'Constitutions of the Air are productive of certain Diseases'. He wondered, however, whether his researches might not reveal something about 'the Nature of the Diseases themselves'.[22] To this end he weighed himself twice daily, weighed the urine he passed and his perspiration, timed his pulse, and numbered and weighed his stools. These and his meteorological observations, which are said to be the first published records of the weather in America, he forwarded to James Jurin, leaving to Jurin the task of interpretation. Jurin seems, however, to have been as unsure about the meaning of these data as was Lining himself. He arranged for the *Philosophical Transactions* to publish parts of the report, for example the summary data that appears here in Table 3.1.[23] Lining could strike certain ratios within the data he reported – observing, for instance, that for the year the quantity of ingesta was 2.02 times heavier than that of urine.[24] But he does not seem to have had anything else in mind than finding ratios embedded in these phenomena.

When Jurin failed in the published report to explain what might be inferred from the tables, Lining wrote again.[25] Somewhat testily he reminded Jurin of the importance of research into the environment–epidemic relationship, and explained the reasons behind the particular experiments he had followed. Are not these matters 'the only *Index* [we have] of the Changes produced in the human Constitution, by the Vicissitudes of the Weather?'[26] Perhaps it would be helpful also to measure the specific gravity of the blood in different diseases, but Lining lacked the necessary instruments. Once again, however, the inferences he drew had to do with relative quantities, and most especially with the pattern of increase and decrease of quantities: 'The mean diurnal Urine in Febr. was increased .07 Parts of what was the mean diurnal Urine in Jan. and was increased .18 Parts of what was the mean diurnal Urine in *March*'.[27] Lining had no mortality or morbidity data to offer, and it is thus difficult to determine why he expected his research to be revealing about disease. Evidently he hoped to establish certain principles about the relationship of ingesta and excreta, which could then serve as a scheme against which to interpret the seasonal alteration of epidemics. But he left Jurin

TABLE 3.1 *Lining's summary of statical data*

Urina est ad Ingesta ut 1 ad	*Perspir. est ad Ingesta ut 1 ad*	*Excret. Alvin. sunt ad Ingest. ut 1 ad*	*Urina est ad Perspir. ut 1 ad*	*Barometri Altitudo*		*Therm. Fabreu. Altitudo.*			*Hygrofcap. Altitudo.*			*Pluvia Quantil*
				Max	*Min.*	*Max.*	*Min.*	*Med.*	*Max.*	*Min.*	*Med.*	
1. 66	2. 71	32. 86	0. 61	30. 40	29. 60	80	34	57	25	4	12	1. 143
1. 85	2. 27	32. 89	0. 82	30. 48	29. 58	83	51	67	14	2	7	1. 092
2. 15	2. 01	34. 61	1. 04	30. 30	29. 90	87	56	74	30	2	9	5. 612
2. 39	1. 75	33. 14	1. 36	30. 28	29. 90	90	66	79	28	5	10	4. 648
3. 07	1. 54	34. 06	1. 99	30. 22	29. 98	91	70	81	30	4	11	3. 013
2. 35	1. 83	30. 75	1. 28	30. 25	29. 95	90	67	77	34	4	12	7. 301
2. 95	1. 53	26. 46	1. 92	30. 36	29. 86	84	56	75	19	6	12	3. 200
2. 03	2. 37	15. 67	0. 85	30. 50	29. 95	73	35	56	33	4	12	1. 255
1. 21	2. 71	30. 08	0. 64	30. 55	29. 73	67	32	52	31	3	14	1. 818
1. 67	2. 77	31. 71	0. 60	30. 58	29. 65	69	21	42	29	3	10	2. 736
1. 62	2. 98	28. 96	0. 55	30. 65	29. 54	63	31	45	40	6	18	4. 492
1. 51	3. 16	36. 82	0. 48	30. 63	29. 88	68	30	46	43	7	16	3. 135
												39. 475

and his readers with an undigested body of information. The things that he had observed and recorded did not reveal any obvious or direct associations with disease.

By studying ingesta and excreta as an index of the cumulative effect of environmental forces on metabolism, however, Lining threatened to complicate further the procedure of the medicine of the environment. Not only did he introduce new phenomena to be measured and examined for correlation, but also he introduced a new class of phenomena, one that could be investigated only by means of procedures of the most tedious sort. Toward the end of the century William Stark revived statical experiments,[28] but in the interim this line of inquiry did not influence environmentalist investigations. Lining was not, however, alone in proposing a new variable not considered by the early environmentalists.

Joseph Raulin suggested the investigation of another phenomenon. Trained at Bordeaux, Raulin set up practice in a small town in Gascony but, on Montesquieu's advice, moved at mid-century to Paris. In time, and through numerous publications, he acquired an international reputation which is reflected in his membership in a number of learned societies. But in 1752 Raulin was a man with some ideas and no substantial reputation. In *Des maladies occasionnées par les promptes et frequentes variations de l'air*, he seized upon an idea already in circulation to begin to build his own reputation.[29]

Raulin's discovery was that, in considering the effect of atmosphere on disease, physicians had been too little attentive to the consequences of sudden and frequent changes in weather conditions. He believed these to be one of the principal causes of illness and chief determinants of proper therapy.[30] Following Arbuthnot and Boyle, Raulin maintained that the atmosphere 'contains vapours, effluvium, and all the particles that detach themselves from bodies and are sufficiently rarefied to float in the atmosphere'.[31] Excessive heat and cold, and excessive humidity are dangerous. It is, nevertheless, the sudden and frequent variation of these things that occasions disease.[32] Such occurrences are common; it is especially fevers that they produce.[33] Raulin therefore regarded barometric pressure as less important, for it is too seldom subject to sharp enough variations to account for the frequency of disease. In this heavily speculative work, attention falls not on weather data, and only infrequently on disease histories. Raulin proposed an hypothesis, but he made no effort to test it. In a longer work published two years later, he discussed things suspended in the atmosphere in more detail and, like Short, identified a great number of forces that may, by adding to the contents of the atmosphere, influence disease. Earthquakes, for example, may cause epidemics through the emanations they add to the air.[34]

Whereas Lining collected metabolic and weather data without a parallel quantity of disease histories, Raulin's 1752 treatise presented disease histories without weather data. By the time they wrote, the interrelatedness of environmental and disease phenomena had been assumed for nearly three-quarters of a century. But it was still an uncommon thing for the several species of data to be gathered simultaneously. A vast body of information was being collected. The physicians who were gathering it demonstrate that they understood the hypothesis of an environment–disease association well enough to see the need to collect data and to see what data to collect. What is curious is that they did not usually see the need to collect simultaneously data on all the variables that they identified as relevant. And if observations were made of all the relevant variables, they were made only for short periods, such as in some of the sources considering the epidemic constitution of a single year or single disease experience. Linig believed he had made an important discovery in learning that the weight of urine passed varied from month to month. But he did not see the need either to publish these tables for several years in succession, to expand the inquiry from a single case (himself) to several cases, or to relate these weights to concurrent diseases.

Thomas Short's long years of observations were undertaken in part, he wrote, in order to test Boyle's hypothesis that 'subterranean Exhalations ascend more copiously' in the spring, when the earth is loosened and the sun is rising toward the perpendicular, than at other times of the year.[35] His researches in the mortality registers seemed to show that more deaths occurred in the spring than in any other season. The data revealed a correlation between deaths and exhalations, and perhaps also between deaths and the 'Rarefaction and Dilation of the Fluids in our Vessels' with 'the Outlets of the Skin not being yet proportionately widened, to give free Vent to the accumulated perspirable Matter'.[36] To notice the parallel occurrence is sufficient; it is the test he had in mind. Short fulfilled his own goal.

In a word, the goal of environmental pathology was to collect data, not to analyse it. The hypothesis was taken to be a theory. This is not an uncommon feature of scientific inquiry in the eighteenth century. Perhaps the group of scientists closest to the environmentalists – both in the data that interested them and in their reading of sources in common – was the demographers. They, too, sought to gather data with as yet a hazy idea about how to use these data to test their assumptions and expectations about population dynamics. Süssmilch believed in the existence of a divine plan, and therefore expected to find a limited number of fixed ratios embedded in population dynamics – one fixed law of the sex ratio at birth, one range of population–mortality ratios according to the density of settlement.[37] Süssmilch therefore was content to gather data in order to compute the ratios embedded in them. Like Lining, he expected this procedure to reveal the implications of the data without requiring further reflection. It is important to notice the degree to which medical statistics relied on political arithmetic for procedures and expectations. Petty's influence sent both demography and medical statistics off in the same direction in terms of the kinds of information sought, the way it was sought, and the great confidence of the researcher that the data collected would be revealing in themselves.

CONCLUSION

'It might be expected, that the science of medicine should, long ago, have arrived to a greater degree of certainty than it has yet attained'.[38] John Millar thus opened his *Observations on the Prevailing Diseases in Great Britain.* Eighteenth-century physicians did not lack the notion of a more efficacious medicine. In their understanding of mortality data, the great divergence between mortality–population ratios from site to site demonstrated a failure of medicine. The statistical techniques of the political arithmeticians were taken over into the medicine of the environment, leading to a search for data and to a certain organisation of those data. The environmentalist wished to collect a large body of observations about features of the habitat and mortality. Only slowly did it become clear that the data sets would have to parallel one another to be useful. Provided with observations, the environmentalist searched for the ratios embedded in them, hoping to discover parallel movements, or the absence of such movement, which would reveal a relationship of cause or at least of influence. To see the ratios was a goal in the medicine of the environment, as it was also in eighteenth-century population studies. That these procedures, which consumed vast amounts of time and energy, did not reveal what was expected of them escaped notice.

4 Epidemiological and Environmental Surveillance: Reasoning About Environmental Pathogens

> This observation confirms what I have been saying, that in cold countries the nervous glands are less expanded.[1]
>
> Montesquieu

John Arbuthnot simultaneously called for the collection of data that would reveal the elements of the environment–disease association, and explained some of the conclusions that could be drawn in advance of the data collection. Later environmentalists collected data, and believed that it pointed up associations. No one seriously doubted the theory of environmental influences upon disease, and physicians who found themselves little interested in this association, such as Boerhaave, did not doubt environmentalism. Rather they concerned themselves preeminently with individual rather than large-group manifestations of disease.

We know already that the hypothesis of an association between environment and disease was accepted before being subjected even to the weak tests that Thomas Short performed on Robert Boyle's theory of emanations,[2] and before parallel data had been gathered in sufficient quantity to allow any comparison of series. In other words, we have discovered that the medicine of the environment was accepted on other grounds than those proposed by its proponents, who called for a test via observation and correlation. Some factors behind this acceptance, such as the powerful support involved in the source of these ideas, in Hippocratic writings, have been identified. Here the issue is those elements of logic and method that led to the assumption that hypothesis had become theory. What to the environmentalist constituted proof, or at least persuasive testimony?

FROM HYPOTHESIS TO THEORY

Short's acceptance of Boyle's idea about subterranean exhalations and emanations – and, more generally, the method Short followed to infer specific environment–disease associations – raise several interesting questions about methodology. These can be approached by a closer examination of Short's writings and by looking more broadly into the literature of environmental pathology at the middle of the eighteenth century. What did physicians like Short mean when they asserted that they intended to base their inferences upon observed phenomena rather than upon existing theories about disease causation? What, more specifically, did these physicians have in mind when they thought of or described the environment–disease association as being correlative? And, I think most intriguing, what arithmetic and statistical techniques were available to be used to explore the correlative relationship that seemed to exist? It is possible that, by asserting a relationship of correlation, the environmentalists anticipated something they could not yet explore, even using the most advanced mathematical techniques of the day. Their failure to clarify the nature of the relationship they assumed to exist may therefore be explained in part by flawed reasoning (i.e., the merely superficial rejection of presupposition), and in part by a failure to grasp the need always to collect data about several or all of the forces and effects presumed to be related to one another. But the explanation may also arise from the simple unavailability of any means to execute the design that, however indeterminantly specified, the environmentalists had in mind.

To take these questions in sequence, what did Sydenham and Short and so many physicians living between them mean by eschewing 'hypotheses' for observation and inference from observation? Sydenham, and in general the environmentalists who followed him, claimed that they would learn effective therapies by accumulating observations of their patients and watching carefully for what was and what was not efficacious.[3] In one sense they were asserting that the process of learning which therapies are effective in which circumstances is unique with each physician, and can be passed on only in the inevitably vague recommendation to be attentive. At the same time, however, Sydenham, Hoffmann, Boerhaave and other devotees of observation expected to derive a lengthening list of aphorisms of the Hippocratic sort. By learning these aphorisms the apprentice physician would narrow the range of what had to be learned from observation.

To the retrospective student, Sydenham seems to have had in mind a process of observing patients and therapies, and later environmentalists a process of observing the environment and epidemics, which would then provide the basis for inferences about relationships between those things. But that second step, the step of drawing inferences from observations, is not clearly explained in the medical literature of the period from the 1660s to 1750. Sydenham, Hoffmann, and Boerhaave took some pains to report how they observed patients, and which therapies they regarded as effective. But they do not reveal how they recognised an effective therapy. All three of them, and physicians in general, continued to blend a selection of so-called heroic treatments – such as bleeding and purging – with medications of which most, like the heroic treatments, do not seem likely to have been beneficial. Theirs was a confusing problem. How could one sort out the patient who recovered despite the application of harmful or useless therapies? In any event, we notice them observing sickness, experimenting with therapies, and selecting some therapies as efficacious. We hear little from them about occasions when a therapy tested and shown beneficial in previous use failed to produce the expected results. We hear little of their therapeutic failures. And we see little scepticism about the range of treatments available, even though our retrospective knowledge persuades us that it should have been difficult to observe any beneficial results from these particular treatments.

In a phrase, these physicians lacked a clear idea of what constitutes an appropriate test of a proposition. If they failed effectively to test prevailing therapies, they were no better placed to evaluate and specify the associations they believed to exist in the environment–disease relationship. The preoccupation of these physicians with accumulating an historical record of the environment or of epidemics is entirely analogous with the preoccupation of the clinicians of that day with building an historical record of illness. Lacking a clear idea of how to relate clinical observations to therapies or the historical record to epidemics and their causes, the physicians saw only vaguely what it was that they needed to observe. On the one hand, they continued to rely on 'hypotheses' – the hypotheses that led to a belief in the efficacy of heroic treatments or the validity of the environment–disease association. On the other hand, they observed both too many things and too few things. Because they did not see clearly how to draw inferences from their observations, they did not see how to distinguish which features of pathogenesis in the patient or the environment needed special attention.

Second, what, more specifically, did the early environmentalists mean when they wrote of correlations or other forms of association between the environment and epidemic disease? For the most part, medical statisticians used the word or the concept of correlation to refer to the simultaneous movement of two or more phenomena – of the seasons of the year and mortality or of specific meteorological phenomena and epidemics. Consider, for example, Short's interpretation of Lining's 'statical Experiments'.[4] In harmony with Lining's expectations, Short found the most important revelations to deal with seasonal ratios of excretions: in the ratios of urine, perspiration, and defecation quantities he discovered what struck him as a reasonable explanation for seasonal variations of dysentery, diarrhoea, and gastrointestinal ailments. The most marked change in these ratios, Lining's data showed, came between summer and autumn, hence Short inferred that in autumn such disorders could be accounted for by that change.[5] As excretory quantities moved upward or downward, the probability of disease changed. In a cloudy or moist season, for instance, diarrhoea would be more common still. The relationship between season and disease could always be clarified if only enough phenomena were considered, until finally one discovered a variable that moved in harmony with the disease. Then the search could be suspended.

Short would thus lengthen the list of phenomena to be observed until every disease movement found its parallel, and explanatory, environmental counterpart. Other environmentalists preferred a shorter list of relevant variables and a more sensitive treatment of their effects. In some cases the cause of an epidemic or endemic disease seemed to be the sustained invariability of a phenomenon, such as the constancy of a wind direction or the prevalence of standing waters, of which Hippocrates had written. For the most part, however, the environmentalists took cause or occasion to lie with variability, and to conceive of the problem in what we can recognise as combinatorial terms. It is not the parallel movement of one disease and one variable or one constant environmental force that is important, but the conjunction of several environmental forces operating jointly and in their joint operation leading to epidemics. Avoidance or being warned depended on an early detection of the signs of this combinatorial variability. Locke and many others too thus looked for the first signs of the change of seasons (the arrival and departure of swallows at Oates) and the first indications of a new atmospheric or environmental constitution (as revealed, for example, by meteorological instruments).

That the data being assessed for simultaneous movement were sometimes defective has already been established. The technique of discovering correlations, we now see, was also defective, since simultaneous movement (or the stillness of one phenomenon and the movement or another) should not by itself have been taken to demonstrate an association of any significance. Aware, like Graunt, of the danger inherent in believing that increased mortality should be thought owing to diminished healthiness rather than to an increase in the number of people at risk, Petty proposed to substitute mean age at death as a technique for finding the most salubrious locale in England. But Petty failed to notice that the populations he was examining were neither stationary nor characterised by identical age structures. Short blundered back into the error of assuming that increased mortality necessarily meant a waxing of the death rate rather than merely of the population at risk, and hazarded 'increased Luxury, Pride, Intemperance, and Debauchery' as the causal forces at work.[6] In other respects, too, such as sloppy arithmetic, Short's statistics look like a regression from Petty's or Graunt's. Nevertheless it was Short who opted for lengthening the list of relevant variables. Only a longer list could provide enough instances of plausible variability or sameness to account for simultaneous epidemics. Short thus added, and added quite substantially, to the scope of the historical record that needed to be accumulated, and to the magnitude of the combinatorial problem facing the epidemiologist.

Major Greenwood shows how much influence Short (or at least Short's portrayal of environment–disease associations) had on British medicine by remarking on how long Short's associations continued to be 'part of the common stock of lay and, perhaps, professional belief'.[7] Outside Britain, Short was seldom cited. But the step he took of adding to the list of variables deemed relevant became inescapable. Because new epidemics of the same disease inevitably occurred in different environmental circumstances, the French, the German, the American, the Italian, and all other environmentalists had to extend their search toward new variables and new combinations. Lining and Raulin added single classes of phenomena to the list of things considered relevant. Others added more than one thing or one class. As the list got longer, the combinatorial possibilities it presented grew more rapidly still. Each new variable resembles a die added to a game of dice: it implied related phenomena (such as Lining's short list of the relevant variables in his meteorostatical tables), and it posed an increasingly complex set of combinatorial problems.

The failure to detect invariable (or at least highly frequent) environment–disease associations did not draw direct comment in eighteenth-century literature. One way to account for this apparent failure to notice the absence of correlations lies with the powerful presuppositions the environmentalists brought to their investigations. Expecting to discover associations between the environment and disease, they did not consider the possibility that such associations do not exist. Nor did they consider the possibility that these associations exist but only in another framework than provided for by environmentalist theory. It is this second thing that we might look for, searching the eighteenth-century sources for suggestions or hints of the existence of intermediaries – microorganisms and vectors – between the environment and disease. Such a search would be relevant to us today and to the suspicion that new theories such as the germ–vector theory find their origins in uneasiness with existing theories.

Here our concern is with eighteenth-century medicine on its own terms, so it is more relevant to ask why the environmentalists failed to notice that the association they believed to exist between the milieu and disease did not, in their terms, exist. Why, as they gathered more and more data about the environment and epidemic disease did not the frequent absence, or the excessive complexity of hypothetical associations, lead to a questioning of the Hippocratic–Sydenham synthesis? Why did physician after physician, to the end of the eighteenth century and well beyond, continue to accept the premise? Much of the answer lies of course with the comfort of habitual patterns of thought. But it is difficult to document or specify what exactly there is in conventional ideas that makes them so resistant to rejection. Here we confront a group of epidemiologists who believed that they were engaged in a new direction of the physician's gaze, in revising and improving medicine in both theory and practice. Here I believe the answer to these questions lies less with the comfort of conventional belief than with the inadequacy of mathematical tools available to puzzle out the terms of the relationships supposed to exist. Lacking mathematical tools adequate to the task of sorting out environment–disease associations, or sorting out the absence of such associations, the epidemiologists should not be expected to have noticed that their presuppositions needed reexamination.

The device of primary use to environmentalism was mathematical expectation as formulated by Pascal and Huygens and discussed by Arbuthnot.[8] The Pascal–Huygens form provided a mathematical technique by means of which the future likelihood of dying from a given cause in a certain place and time could be estimated by discovering the historical ratio of deaths from that cause in proportion to deaths from all causes in that place and for an analogous time. In this formulation, the statistical investigation of mortality or of any other phenomenon, and the projection of future trends on the basis of historical experience, counted on the law of large numbers. According to this law, the margin of error in any statistical sample (or historical record) may be presumed to diminish as the number of cases in the sample (or record) increases.[9] This is, therefore, a process in which the researcher seeks a sufficiently large segment of a total population to represent the experience of the total population, rather than a small but random sample. How large the segment of a total population should be remains an unknown. The development of random sampling has evaded this issue for many researchers, who have access to a total population and can take a random sample from it. But the issue remains germane to historical research in which information is seldom available about total populations, and the historian often wants to know what portion – 10 per cent, 30 per cent, 50 per cent? – of the total must be represented before a satisfactory degree of accuracy may be achieved.

For the eighteenth-century epidemiologist the law of large numbers was a new discovery – a principle worked out in the seventeenth century and gradually disseminated.[10] Many demographers and environmentalists had no appreciation of it, and many others had only an intuitive appreciation. But the thrust of the medicine of the environment as of science in general was clearly influenced by the law of large numbers. Environmentalists sought to gather as much data as they could about mortality and environmental characteristics. The longer and larger the historical record, the most content the physician was that it would affirm the environment–disease association and reveal its specific features.

Writing in 1781, William Black put matters in this way:

> To form useful Tables of the ratio of mortality at various ages, to determine upon the relative havock by different diseases, upon the general effects of seasons, climates, and situations, of diet, drink, modern luxuries, and new manners, we should . . . take in an interval of many years, and include large groups of mankind.[11]

More than a century after the formulation in the 1650s and 1660s of a mathematics of expectation relying on the law of large numbers, the medical statistician continued to rely upon the collection of large bodies of data. What we must notice about this testimony from Black, a highly capable statistician, is the emphasis given the accumulation of data. Because the technique of taking a random sample remained undiscovered, and because no progress had been made in deciding how large a non-random sample must be in order to provide a satisfactory degree of accuracy, the statistician searched inevitably for more and more data. And if the vast body of data that one researcher, such as Black, gathered did not reveal the thing being searched for, the most advanced statistical techniques in use suggested a search for still more data.

In the first place, therefore, the medicine of the environment had to build an historical record about the phenomena deemed relevant, and in the second it had to keep adding observations until they revealed the things being searched for. When the record showed fixed associations, or when an entire population had been observed, the accumulation could be suspended. But fixed associations were never discovered, and entire populations could not be observed because the physician and his allies lacked the means to do so, and because those agencies which attempted something of the sort, such as the compilers of the London bills of mortality, failed adequately to execute their task.

In the reasoning of eighteenth-century population theory, the search into population dynamics was expected to reveal fixed ratios, or a fixed range of ratios, within demographic phenomena. The search should thus reveal a range of mortality–population ratios for the various densities and salubrities of settlement. The search should thus reveal a fixed ratio of the sexes at birth. Sometimes this quest for the natural laws of demography was productive. Arbuthnot discovered that male births regularly exceed female births in large groups, and later demographers gathered more data until they could hypothesise a sex ratio close to that accepted by present-day historical demography: twenty-one males per twenty females. At other times the search revealed no fixed ratios, or no fixed and reasonably narrow range of ratios. In mortality data, for example, the population statistician found a wide divergence between urban and rural mortality ratios and (because differences in age structure were not noticed) an even wider ratio within cities or the countryside. In any event, the demographer was researching phenomena which, we can see in retrospect, often possess fixed or narrow ranges of proportion. There are, for example, certain modal life expectancies to be found in eighteenth-century populations.

In environmental pathology, however, essentially inconstant phenomena were being investigated. Further investigations produced more rather than less diversity. And, in the eighteenth-century approach to statistical analysis, the discovery of more diversity demanded additional investigations. In the interim the environmentalists speculated about correlations. But they felt obliged to continue to accumulate data, as we see from Black's call toward the end of the eighteenth century, after more than a century of data collection. What is to be noticed is that it was the epidemiologists who knew the most of advanced statistical techniques, who had an explicit grasp of the law of large numbers, who felt inclined to press for more data. The best informed application of mathematical expectation as understood in the eighteenth century thus led the environmentalist away from rather than toward any scepticism about the general proposition of a direct environment–disease relationship. This is evident in Black's vast compilation of data. It is evident also in the yet more vast attempt organized by Vicq d'Azyr to collect data about the climate and disease in France. It is evident in general in the medicine of the environment in the latter decades of the century, a medicine in the hands of Finke in Germany, of Currie in the United States, of Van den Bosch in the Dutch Netherlands, of Thiéry in Spain, and of other physicians in other places. The medicine of the environment never suffered, in the eighteenth century, any general or abiding scepticism about the assumptions that lay behind it.

LOGIC

If mathematics led the medical statistician away from scepticism, so did logic. The logical device the eighteenth-century physician used to infer the validity or the reasonableness of an idea was the device of reasoning from analogy or, to be more specific, inductive analogy.[12] To the environmentalist as to biologists and to many scientific and philosophical thinkers stretching back to medieval Christian theologians, including the contagion theorist Fracastoro,[13] one means of showing the truth of a proposition was to point to analogical relationships, to search for similarities believed to exist between objects in nature and objects contrived by man.[14] By such means the theologian had established as a universal principle the hierarchy of things in the spiritual realm by arguing from the analogy of a hierarchy of things in human society. This form of reasoning is common also in classical philosophy, which helps explain its use in early modern medicine.[15] The Birmingham physician Richard Pearson, doubtful about the medicinal uses of gases, thus reconsidered, 'saw analogy on its side; and after he had bestowed further attention upon it, he saw it was supported by facts'.[16]

A famous case of analogical reasoning to reach inferences is provided by Montesquieu,[17] whose specific example of how analogical reasoning leads to reliable conclusions seemed persuasive to such physicians as William Falconer:[18]

> I have observed the outermost part of a sheep's tongue, where, to the naked eye, it seems covered with papillae. On these papillae I have discerned through a microscope small hairs, or a kind of down; between the papillae were pyramids shaped towards the ends like pincers. Very likely these pyramids are the principal organ of taste.
>
> I caused the half of this tongue to be frozen, and observing it with the naked eye I found the papillae considerably diminished: even some rows of them were sunk into their sheath. The outermost part I examined with the microscope, and perceived no pyramids. In proportion as the frost went off, the papillae seemed to the naked eye to rise, and with the microscope the miliary glands began to appear.
>
> This observation confirms what I have been saying, that in cold countries the nervous glands are less expanded: they sink deeper into their sheaths, or they are sheltered from the action of external objects; consequently they have not such lively sensations.
>
> In cold countries they have very little sensibility for pleasure; in temperate countries, they have more; in warm countries, their sensibility is exquisite. As climates are distinguished by degrees of latitude, we might distinguish them also in some measure by those of sensibility. I have been at the opera in England and in Italy, where I have seen the same pieces and the same performers; and yet the same music produces such different effects on the two nations: once is so cold and phlegmatic, and the other so lively and enraptured, that it seems almost inconceivable.

Cold temperatures produce diminished sensibility in ovine taste organs; therefore a cold climate produces diminished sensibility in living organisms in general. This technique, which allows a wide and untestable range of inferences from analogy, constituted one of the fundamental tools of reasoning in the eighteenth century.

To an important extent statistics as practised by the environmentalists amounts to a numerative form of reasoning from analogy. In the environmentalist's numerative image of the world one could expect to find a pattern in things, and one could expect to find that pattern in the shape of fractions and ratios representing statements about elementary forms. When, for instance, in human births males were discovered to exceed females, the statistician uncovered an elementary form. The numerative statement of the imbalance, at Graunt's fourteen: thirteen or at the narrower ratio eventually reached at twenty-one: twenty, is a precise description that not only affirms the existence of laws but also reveals the terms of one law.

Whereas on the one hand the ratios derived by statisticians represented numerative forms for discussing phenomena subject to analysis by reasoning from analogy, on the other mathematical expectation furnished a way to infer proofs from analogical reasoning that depended directly on numerative descriptions of phenomena.[19] Huygens, in the textbook on mathematical expectation that Arbuthnot translated into English, explained that the equation $A/B = C/D$ (where A is the number of historical cases of deaths from a particular cause and B the number of all known deaths from all causes) establishes the likelihood of any current death (D) being from the same cause (C). Huygens also explained that this procedure may be used to estimate the future proportion or likelihood of any phenomenon for which satisfactory historical data can be found. Huygens would use the historical record on given phenomena to predict the future proportions of those phenomena. But the medical and environmental statisticians failed to distinguish between mathematical expectation's statement of equality between historical and future ratios of the *same* phenomenon, and the assertion of an analogical relationship within the historical record of *different* phenomena.

An argument from analogy provided the logical foundations for the medicine of the environment: environmental factors influence the temperament and character of peoples; by analogy it follows that the same factors influence health.[20] Upon that premise, and using a qualitative or a quantitative form for expressing ideas about specific analogies, the environmentalists posited the existence of hundreds, even thousands, of specific analogies. For example, Lining detected an inverse relationship between urine and perspiration, according to which one increased in warm weather as the other diminished. By reasoning from analogy, this observation could be used to infer the cause of, or the occasion for, diseases occurring at the same time as a change of seasons and a shift in the urine–perspiration ratio. The numerative form of reasoning from analogy did not require that phenomena shift in the same direction, as this example from Lining's work shows. It also did not require that things in both sides of the analogy-equation change at all. Consider the permutations among a long list of variables among which change may or may not be significant, and among which significant changes may occur in opposite as well as similar directions. The potential for drawing analogous inferences knew hardly any bounds. Reasoning from analogy added further to an already imposing set of combinatorial possibilities.

Finally along this line it should be noticed that the quantities presumed to be relevant in describing simultaneous movement in analogical relationships were expressed in the form of annals or tables. The earliest example of a graphical presentation of such data is usually held to have occurred in a 1669 letter from Christiaan Huygens to his brother Lodewijk.[21] Christiaan wanted to show how Graunt's partly conjectural tables of survivors at certain ages out of a population of a hundred might be used to estimate survivorship at ages not mentioned, and to solve other problems. But the expression of such data in graphical form did not catch on until the end of the eighteenth century, as we have already noticed. How the people studying the annals and tables or merely the prose accounts of statistical data construed those data is not apparent. Did they develop in their mind's eye graphical images? Did they seek or find any technique for 'seeing' the associations embedded in the annals, tables, or prose accounts? I cannot answer these questions, but I can make one useful remark. Environmentalists usually expected associations to be immediate rather than lagged.[22] However they pictured the raw data available to them, they looked for relationships that would show up quickly. In this way the range of potential environment–disease associations was narrowed from what it might have been. But the narrowing takes on the quality of an oversight, for the relevance of lagged effects was not considered and rejected by most environmentalists, it was merely left unmentioned.

Nevertheless we can find growing confidence in the tabular arrangement of data in the mere increasing frequency of tables, such as in Francis Clifton's *Tabular Observations* of weather, disease, therapy, and outcome, and the tables compiled by the agents of the Société royale de médecine in France. Clifton, physician to the Prince of Wales, asserted his confidence in the tabular arrangement of data by writing: 'Nor will I ever write upon any subject, as a Physician, for which I have not *Tabular Authority*'.[23] On the one hand, Clifton helped foster use of a scheme for arranging information with obvious advantages over random recall or prose statistical narratives. On the other hand, he attributed to that scheme an authority which it does not possess. Arranging data in the form of a table of course does nothing to interpret those data, yet one finds in the eighteenth-century literature an exaggerated confidence in what the tabular form did or would reveal.[24]

Although they assumed that analogous relationships could be detected by examining historical records of environmental and medical phenomena, the environmentalists did not concentrate on discovering analogies. As Locke had explained by way of justifying the meteorological observations he had made, 'many things relating to the Air, Winds, Health, Fruitfulness, *&c.* might by a sagacious man be collected from them, and several Rules and Observations concerning the extent of Winds and Rains, &c. be in time establish'd'.[25] The confidence felt in the ultimate powers of reasoning from analogy provided another reason for concentrating on the collection rather than the interpretation of data. For one thing, medical statisticians (like their counterparts studying population) believed that the detection of quantities and ratios between and among phenomena was itself a species of analysis. More generally, however, the device of reasoning from analogy left the focus of attention on discovering and detailing things analogous. The analogy itself did not require development because it was obvious. Locke, Lining, and the other environmentalists counted on 'sagacious men' to see things that were obvious, even if they themselves did not.

APPLIED ENVIRONMENTAL MATHEMATICS

All the labour of the environmentalists was not devoted to the compilation of data. Several times I have mentioned examples of intuitive inferences. Now I want to turn to some examples of the way in which environmentalists used the historical record they were compiling to draw conclusions about specific elements of the environment–disease association.

Graunt had provided a numerative demonstration for things already believed on non-numerative grounds. He thus asked whether cities are less healthy than rural areas, compared mortality and estimated living populations in some sample cities and rural areas, and concluded that cities were unhealthy, especially for infants and children. People already believed this to be true, and their belief was grounded in experience. Graunt merely demonstrated the proportions of something already known, showing how to use numbers as adjectives and nouns with a greater capacity than qualitative terms for reflecting shades of difference.

The test that confirmed accepted opinion might also undermine opinion or belief. The Dutch physician Cornelis Bontekoe showed how this might be so in 1683 by using the same technique as Graunt to discover whether climacterics – years within the life cycle of exceptionally heavy mortality – could be affirmed from mortality data. Popular belief held that the ages sixty-three and eighty-one were especially dangerous. The idea of the climacteric had been criticised in 1646 by Thomas Browne, who considered at length the magical powers ascribed to certain numbers, in this instance seven and nine. Browne expressed doubt about the existence of climacterics because of misgivings about such evidence, and because of the unreliability of reported accounts of the deaths of famous people at age 63.[26] To him, scepticism was warranted because the reasons for believing in climacteric years were not convincing.

Graunt introduced, and Bontekoe followed, a different technique. The Dutch physician rejected the controversial idea of climacteric years because, looking at mortality data, he found that few members of a birth cohort survived to age 63, but that of those who did, most lived for some time thereafter.[27] Bontekoe rejected the idea, not because the evidence for it was not sufficiently persuasive but because he looked for (and found) convincing evidence against it. In this way statistical analysis as pioneered by Graunt substantially enhanced the opportunity for testing propositions and clarifying inferences.

For the most part it was upon clarifying inferences rather than testing propositions that the environmentalists focused. Lining thus sought, by deriving ratios of bodily excretions by season, to lay the basis for general laws about the environment–disease association, which laws would take the form of comparatively small shifts identifiable best in numbers because of the power of numbers to allow an infinite degree of differentiation. Nevertheless, the literature occasionally contains a test of existing propositions. An example is to be found in the researches of the physician John Millar, who was a contemporary of but should not be confused with the philosophic historian of the same name. Examining the mortality research of Richard Price and Thomas Percival, Millar constructed a table of the ratio of the annual number of deaths in certain locales to the estimated living population, which he used then to draw inferences about the efficacy of certain treatments and the general efficacy of eighteenth-century medicine. Let us take a sample of his mortality–population ratios, and see what he had to say about them:[28]

London	1:20
Vienna	1:19.5
Berlin	1:26.5
Northampton	1:26
Shrewsbury	1:26
Darwin	1:56
Eastham	1:35
British campaign in Germany, 1759	1:16
British campaign in Germany, 1760	1:8
British campaign in Germany, 1761	1:6

> From this Table it appears that in London and other large towns, where few are sick without medical assistance, nearly one-twentieth of the inhabitants die annually, and in the army, during actual service, when all the sick are attended by physicians, the mortality is still greater. But in other places where diseases are often left to their natural course they prove much less fatal.

Millar discovered some reasons for doubting the efficacy of medical assistance.

He looked also at the London bills of mortality to discover the efficacy of treatments of fevers. Under Boerhaave's influence physicians had followed a regimen of profuse bleeding of fever patients, which Millar claimed would explain the doubling in the numbers of fever deaths reported in the bills. As doses of the Peruvian bark (cinchona or quinine) were substituted for bleeding, the numbers of fever deaths diminished to a level below that existing before Boerhaave's influence had been felt.[29]

These are not, of course, fair tests of the relationship between access to physicians or particular therapies and recovery from sickness, or of the proposition that mortality increases with the incidence of medical attention. Millar acknowledged that other variables were at work. Nevertheless he used such tests as these to bring under general scrutiny some aspects of accepted medical opinion in his day.

What should we notice about this investigation? We should notice, first, that eighteenth-century statistical methods contained defects, some acknowledged at the time and some unacknowledged. Millar might have been even more dubious than he was about mortality–population ratios suggesting a mortality rate as low as 15 per 1 000 per annum in one locale. In any event, Millar saw how to use the statistical techniques of his day to devise a test of some interesting propositions, and recognised that the tests did not have much force. The second thing we should notice here is the conclusion that Millar drew: the relationship of these phenomena is not yet clear; additional information must be gathered. In the meantime Millar wondered about the apparent variability of the environment–disease association. Should the list of ailments believed to be caused by atmospheric forces be shortened? Millar emerged uncertain: 'Though many diseases occur in every season, and in all the various vicissitudes of weather, which do not seem to spring from the qualities of the air, yet it is certain pleurisies, peripneumonies, and other inflammations of the chest . . . are sometimes occasioned by a sudden change from mild weather to rigid frost, accompanied with hail, snow, and storms, and with north and north-easterly winds'.[30]

Millar tested a few propositions. William Black sought in 1781 to inaugurate a general statistical examination of the environment–disease association, and of the influence of non-naturals as a whole upon health. This project would be formed into 'the science of Medical Arithmetick and Universal Prognosticks'.[31] In the process, while criticising the data available to him, Black affirmed the superior healthiness of rural areas, yet detected that some epidemics are less frequently fatal in cities than in villages. This latter finding he explained by suggesting a higher level of resistance or seasoning among city dwellers, an idea others had had before him, and by claiming that environmental factors might play a role. The air of cities 'is charged with a load of smoke, and other heterogeneous vapours' which are ill suited to conduct disease.[32] Like Millar, Black saw medicine as standing yet on the brink of a great leap forward in data collection. Only more data would reveal the answers that for the moment could not be given.

CONCLUSION

The curious issue that intrigues is the failure of these physicians to become sceptical about the validity of the environment–disease hypothesis as stated by Sydenham and his associates. Why, especially in the face of variable rather than fixed relationships between environmental phenomena and epidemic disease, did the physician not wonder about the theory, or at least about the form of the theory? The answer to this question we have found in the great complexity of the combinatorial problem posed by an expanding list of variables deemed relevant, in the primitive nature of statistical tools, and in the false assurance of reasoning from analogy. Everything combined to point even the sceptical environmentalist, like James Millar, toward collecting more data.

In retrospect we can see that the association believed by the eighteenth-century physician to exist between the environment and epidemic disease did not exist. Now we can acknowledge both that this belief was general in Europe at that time, and that it was held for what seemed to be sufficient reasons. That is to say, our investigation into patterns of thought reveals that neither medicine nor its ancillary fields, including statistics, stood close to a breakthrough in understanding epidemics. Environmentalism was informed thought. The hypothesis seemed to have become a theory even though, as we see now, it had hardly been tested. It became a theory because of the strong traditions behind it, and because medical inquiry and medical logic failed to produce significant countervailing evidence.

To see these things is to understand the strength of the

environmentalists' conviction. Even if we cannot be misled by that conviction, even if today we admit the general relevance of the environment to disease but focus most of our attention on causes against which the physician or the public health authority has more power to react, we must admit also that the eighteenth-century physician faced a different problem. Medicine was not efficacious or – if one takes the most generous view possible toward eighteenth-century therapies – it had exceedingly modest beneficial effects. In such circumstances it made perfect sense for physicians to direct their attention toward the environment. In man's habitat, as in food and drink, the physician's gaze fell upon something tangible that could be influenced.

5 Avoidance and Prevention of Epidemics

> Once sufficiently ascertained, are these harmful substances indestructible?
>
> Baumes

> in order to correct the deleterious dispositions of localities.[1]
>
> *Encyclopédie méthodique*

ENVIRONMENTAL ENGINEERING IN THEORY

The idea that epidemic diseases arise from, or are caused by, forces in the environment characterised most epidemiological thinking in eighteenth-century Europe. We have explored the idea itself, and the scientific actions that this idea (and the assumptions and techniques associated with it) prompted. The epidemiologist sought to gather observations under an unchallenged expectation that the observations would reveal the form of the association. This search did not produce either verified environmentalist propositions, or general scepticism about the environment–disease association. It did produce, however, a number of speculations and assertions about specific features of the association, and a number of conclusions about the kind of public health action that would be efficacious in avoiding or preventing large-group manifestations of disease.

At the heart of these speculations and conclusions lies an ambition not entirely new to eighteenth-century medicine, but new in the generality and the intensity with which it was held. According to this ambition, it will be more useful to try to control disease at its source than to wait for the stage at which the only reaction must be therapy. In this scheme the physician's gaze shifted from the individual patient to the patient's habitat, and the physician's attention was diverted from Sydenham's concern – efficacious therapy – to the problem of determining those modifications of the habitat that would deter or elude the onset of epidemic disease. In one direction the medicine of the environment prompted the notion of disrupting the environment–disease association by moving people away from habitats deemed unhealthy – the quarantine of the pathogenic site rather than of the diseased individual. In another direction, this medicine promoted certain ideas about altering the habitat to make it healthier. The first remedy the physician encouraged upon his patients, or urged as a general treatment for the uncommonly sickly locale. The second remedy the physician urged upon governments and public spirited individuals as a treatment for the locale itself, or for some temporary features of it. In an address in 1802 to the Philadelphia Medical Society, Charles Caldwell explained some measures that needed adoption:

> We can remove from around our habitations the putrefying recrements of organized bodies. . . . Further, we can erect our dwellings on elevated situations, defend them from the exhalations of millponds and neighboring marshes by interposing ranges of trees, and, by means of flannel clothing, protect our persons from the changes of the weather. Nor is this all. We can substitute vegetables for part of the animal food which we now consume, malt liquor and cider for our high wines and ardent spirits, and, in all other respects, live in conformity to the genius of our climate.[2]

Every environmentalist provided a unique list of the measures to be adopted, for each list was intended to refer to the specific problems of the locale in which the physician practised. Time-worn recommendations, such as Hippolytus Guarinonius' 1610 proposal that the streets and squares of cities be widened to improve perflation – the movement of air – joined new ideas, such as the notion of promoting drainage projects for their public health advantages. To these were added ideas made feasible by eighteenth-century technological innovations, or by the leaps of imagination of the eighteenth-century approach to improving man and man's environment. Caldwell explained that the things he proposed

> fall within the sphere of our power, and it is no less our duty than our interest to attain them. Such an issue would contribute equally to individual health and happiness, and to the prosperity, strength, and aggrandisement of our country. Let us then, like Cadmus of Tyre, wage a war of extermination with these Hydras of disease, that our posterity may live in security from their ravages. The voice of patriotism combines with that of nature and of reason, to urge and animate us in the important enterprize.

These were strong words for an audience of Caldwell's day. Their intensity reveals that a sense of expectation, of standing at the cutting edge of a campaign to conquer disease, remained strong at the end of the eighteenth century.

Let us examine more closely the measures that Caldwell and other physicians proposed to take, and focus our attention especially on four great feats of environmental engineering. Three of these – drainage, lavation, and ventilation – we encountered first in the writings of British environmentalists late in the seventeenth and early in the eighteenth century. These three, and the fourth – reinterment – we encountered in continental environmentalism. Two things distinguish these four measures from the large list of things proposed by someone. In the first place, these measures seemed to eighteenth-century physicians to have a general utility, and so they stand out from the larger body of proposals made to improve the healthiness of specific locales. Second, these measures seemed clearly within the range of things possible: no leap of imagination was required to see their implementation.

Drainage

To the environmentalist one particular configuration seemed consistently to coincide with certain epidemics, and more generally with high mortality and morbidity rates. The low-lying, damp, and often fetid region within and adjacent to swamps and bogs – 'these arsenals of death' – appeared to signal not the highest form of danger, such as might account for plague epidemics, but a more insidious threat to public health.[3] The association of the swamp with disease was not a new idea, but an old notion that received new emphasis whenever the theory of environmental influence upon disease was reasserted. Boyle's notion of emanations gave this idea a revised form, for it hypothesised that standing water may emit, and the air may hold and disseminate, unspecified particles that transmit disease. To the Montpellier physician J. B. T. Baumes, 'the existence of marshy miasmas, and the power they have to propagate intermittent and remittent fevers is at present incontrovertibly beyond doubt'.[4] 'If any Stranger tarries long in boggy Places, and is exposed to a thick Air, within a very few Days he certainly falls sick'.[5] Lancisi's idea of animate vectors such as mosquitoes carrying pathogenic fluids was thus neglected in favor of his hypothesis of an inanimate means of transmission in which swamps produce malaria because they give off emanations transmitted by the atmosphere. Baumes added that the virulence of these miasmas is indicated by their odour.[6]

Rather than merely iterating an old association between standing water and disease, the environmentalist sought a means to disrupt the causal mechanism at work. What is the malleable feature of the swamp? It is standing water, which is open to hydraulic engineering, to drainage.

In the latter decades of the seventeenth century the idea of drainage also was not new. But the environmentalist provided new reasons for undertaking it. Whereas earlier advocates had favoured drainage chiefly as a means of opening new arable land, the environmentalist cited both economic and public health objectives.[7] The *Journal oeconomique* in an issue of 1762, on the eve of a campaign directed by the royal government in France, urged drainage of the Pontine marshes in Italy both for the economic utility of such improvements and because drainage would destroy 'the source of the noxious exhalations that corrupt the air of the most pleasant and fertile plain in Europe'.[8] Or, to give only one more of many possible examples, the curé of Pérols reported a population at one-third its former level after the appearance of paludous areas. The restoration of the canal system of the region returned the population to its former strength and good health.[9]

Between Sydenham and Vicq d'Azyr this form of environmental modification for preventive purposes became a cry not only of the environmentalists but also in general of the proponents of improving man and man's milieu. In the American colonies the loyalist and physician Cadwallader Colden seems to have been the first to discuss this particular association. Citing Lancisi as his source, Colden attributed an epidemic fever that broke out in New York City in 1741 to stagnant waters. Specifically intermittent fever might be prevented by drainage projects or by other means, such as fully submerging marshy areas.[10] By the end of the eighteenth century the utility of drainage seemed in the United States to be commonplace wisdom. Benjamin Rush cited it as one of several modifications of habitat that could prevent the 'bilious and intermitting fevers in Pennsylvania'.[11] Rush attributed the heightened morbidity of 1784 and 1785 to wet spring seasons which 'left a large and extensive surface of moist ground exposed to the action of the sun, and of course to the generation and exhalation of febrile miasmata'.[12] He objected in particular to the construction of mill ponds without taking adequate precautions – periodic clearing and planting trees between such ponds and human habitations, the trees acting as obstructions to the passage of air laden with noxious substances and as cleansers.[13]

At the very end of the century William Currie, concerned specifically with the problem of intermittent fevers, investigated the mechanism making marshy sites so harmful.[14] One line of inquiry taken in this quest had searched into the properties of air. From that had come several ideas about the particular gas or gases given off by swamps and by the animal and vegetable matter putrefying in them. Currie surveyed this research and concluded that the noxious force was not miasmic or any particular gas, but a deficiency of a gas – oxygen – within the air over and around swampy sites. The problem of the swamp, therefore, is the want of a proper mixture of gases, which itself is owing to animal and vegetable decay and putrefaction and to the lack of circulation. As preventive measures Currie pointed vaguely to chemical means of inhibiting putrefaction. But he dismissed them as expensive and impractical. More appropriate would be drainage, filling, and cultivation. By 1799, when these recommendations were made, these were old ideas for improving the healthiness of the American habitat.[15]

In Europe, too, the public health efficacy of drainage came generally to be acknowledged during the eighteenth century. Thomas Short recommended it as a measure whose effects could be demonstrated in his tables of mortality and meteorology.[16]

The Swiss demographer Jean-Louis Muret found that parishes with extensive areas of marshland had higher mortality rates than the hilly districts of the Vaud.[17] That particular finding seemed conclusive proof to Richard Price, the English Nonconformist who supported the American rebels and, among many activities, contributed significantly to the early development of actuarial mathematics.[18]

From France, however, came the most thorough case in favour of drainage. In a general plan for the improvement of the monarchy, the vicomte de La Maillardière identified swamps and marshes as detrimental to agriculture, trade, and the well-being of the kingdom in all respects.[19] La Maillardière, who had read widely in the literature of environmentalism, believed that the source of infection lay not in the air but in the water of the swamp.[20] As corrective, he recommended massive drainage projects on the Prussian model, to be sponsored by the French monarchy, for the execution of which he devised detailed plans.[21] In a time of peace, which was nearing in 1782 when La Maillardière published, royal financing for public works projects seemed feasible. Others agreed. In 1786 Jean Baptiste Banau and François Turben appealed to the estates of Languedoc to adopt a variety of drainage and hydraulic improvements in order to moderate the effects of epidemics in the province.

These are but a few examples of the confidence eighteenth-century epidemiologists felt in the efficacy of drainage. They establish merely that this specific measure for reforming the environment was frequently and widely endorsed. Before turning to the question of implementation, let us consider the other principal measures of environmental modification.

Lavation

Turning their gaze toward the milieu of disease, the environmentalists noticed that the stench of putrefaction proceeds not merely from swamps and bogs but also from a number of other sites in man's habitat. Stench seemed to be the most obvious sign of disease-ridden circumstances within the habitat, and thus more readily recognisable than the complex of meteorological and environmental forces believed to occasion specific diseases. A gaze more attentive to disease in the individual might have prompted more concern with personal cleanliness, but personal hygiene remained a matter of infrequent concern in the eighteenth century. The epidemiologist's preoccupation lay with large-group diseases, and thus it was the cleanliness of site that seemed most intriguing. Here too an idea of great antiquity – the notion that some connection exists between urban drainage and public health – came to be pressed into service anew.[22]

Just as Price was persuaded of the 'insalubrity of marshy situations' by Muret's data from the Vaud, so the environmentalist tested the association between cleansed and uncleansed sites by proposing to compare mortality between locales drained and cleansed by natural means and unlavated sites. From the English town of Chester, situated on a porous rock promontory, the physician John Haygarth reported unusual longevity, which he explained as owing in part to the natural draining and cleansing of the streets by rain, and the regular lavation of Chester's natural subterranean drainage system by tidal action. In consequence the town was free of 'stagnant moisture and putrefaction'.[23]

Fortuitous instances of natural lavation seemed to prove the efficacy of man-made improvements that would have the same effects. So, too, did the comparison of thoroughly with only mildly putrescent sites. The general filth of eastern Mediterranean cities thus sufficed to explain why they suffered more frequent epidemics than did European cities. Frank argued also that cleanliness of site explained how the Dutch combated the effects of living in an epidemic-prone habitat.[24] The environmentalist thus endorsed the effort to build drainage facilities, and to make such hydraulic improvements that filthy urban sites might regularly be flushed and their refuse carried off.

Lavation constituted the urban counterpart of the drainage of standing waters: it would flush not the swamp but the stench-laden refuse and puddles of the urban environment. Human contact with disease-causing substances and their emanations would thereby be diminished, although usually by flushing these things out of the city and into streams and rivers rather than by steps to impede the process of decay and mephitis. Lavation demanded no modification in the behaviour of city-dwellers, whose refuse casually disposed of in public by-ways created a large part of the problem of decay and putrefaction. It merely suggested an extended area of responsibility for municipal government. The task of public authorities would no longer be limited, in the most active city, to the disposal of human waste, such as urban inhabitants of the Austrian Netherlands did by selling night soil to farmers for fertiliser. It would extend to social infrastructure improvements, such as the construction of a means to bring water into the city in sufficient quantity, and to release it with sufficient force, to flush away the urban detritus of man and nature.

That government should play a role in cleansing the urban environment was an old idea. Keen interest in public action to collect and dispose of refuse may be found in a number of Renaissance Italian and German cities.[25] But seventeenth-century examinations of mortality by site (those of Graunt and Petty especially) detected that the city was still an unhealthy location. In a variety of metaphors the urban locale came to be condemned as a consumer of lives, a cause of population decline. The environmentalists took over this view of the city, but proposed a counterattack via lavation. To Frank 'towns contain in concentration . . . all the causes of uncleanliness which are only very dispersed in the country'.[26] But the city can be made as healthy as the countryside.

Lavation constituted a central method of modifying the urban habitat, but the environmentalists proposed many measures to treat this manifestation of the pathogenic milieu. Their programme extended to a broad agenda of measures to make the city clean and orderly, measures grouped together in the eighteenth century under the heading of 'police'. Frank thus argued for municipal intervention to prevent the pollution of streams and rivers in the same passage where he proclaimed the utility of flushing human dwellings periodically with flowing waters.[27] Casting about for ideas, Frank noticed that in Hamburg refuse was daily carted outside the city. He noticed also that several German towns contained public latrines which were lacking in other places and countries where, he believed, human waste was deposited casually in the streets. And he discovered towns where polluting manufactures and refuse pits had been relocated outside of and downwind from human settlement. These and many other measures he proposed as means of policing the environment.[28] The distinctive feature about Frank's programme is the role assigned in it to public authorities, and to a new cooperation between them and physicians interested in public health. Frank imagined a world in which emperors and kings, Joseph II of Austria, and later Napoleon and Alexander I of Russia, would heed the advice of their public health advisers. The motto of the eighteenth-century populationist – that the strength of the state lies in the number of its citizens – he revised: the wealth of the state lies in the health of its subjects.[29]

Although it is especially Germany that is renowned as the land where the proponents of improvement focused on this particular style of action, Frank's ideas and the related proposals of other proponents of policing reforms found support elsewhere also. Jean Emmanuel Gilibert, author of *L'anarchie médicinale* and critic of the French medical establishment, called for a restoration of preventive medicine in France by similar means.[30] Other French hygienists explained how to pave and cleanse streets,[31] to provide fresh water for the city, to shift polluting industries away from densely settled areas. One of the great unrealised projects of the French old regime was to install companies that would make a profit from collecting and disposing of urban refuse.[32] Neither in France nor elsewhere was there any shortage of ideas for cleansing the urban environment.

Ventilation

To the environmentalist one of the intriguing elements of the Hippocratic tradition lay in the paradox that the 'air is the father of human life and of human diseases'.[33] As explained in the *Journal oeconomique* in a 1764 article luridly entitled 'Effets terribles de la putréfaction', 'air corrupted by putrefaction is the most fatal of all causes of illness'.[34] To be cleansed and purified, air must circulate. Thereby it is constantly freshened, constantly renewed after respiration or contact with putrescent substances.

To buttress this case, the anonymous article in the *Journal oeconomique* cited the researches of the environmentalist physician John Pringle. But Pringle was only one of several scientists whose investigations of the environment confirmed the old suspicion that stench is a sign of disease-conducive properties in the atmosphere and, more specifically, that the degree of stench corresponds to the degree of harmfulness.[35]

One line of research into this problem sought distinctions among categories of 'putrescible substances'. The lexicographer

Noah Webster, following the lead of the physicians Rush and Currie, believed the putrescence of animal and human faeces to be not nearly as harmful as that of rotting vegetable refuse, which he would have buried or thrown into the sea.[36] With complete seriousness, in contrast to Swift's treatise on the varieties of excrement, Webster reported the results of recent research on the air within privies.[37] It is, he said, less noxious than people believe, which shows that the association between stench and unhealthiness is more complex than it has been imagined to be.[38] In the city of Metz, Michel du Tennetar compiled a topography of odours.[39] But these were fine distinctions, so many more variables in an already imposing combinatorial problem. More generally the environmentalist of the second half of the eighteenth century was concerned to condemn all malodorous sites and all particularly acute stenches, and to show how to relieve them and to inhibit their contribution to the onset of epidemics.

For the site whose stench could not be removed by drainage or lavation, or by chemical treatment with vinegar vapours or hydrochloric acid,[40] the environmentalist proposed ventilation. This was not, of course, a practical step for any open site, where the treatment of preference would be to remove the source of mephitis. Where ventilation would be effective would be the closed area – the dwelling, meeting hall, ship, hospital, prison, any place where people gathered in an enclosed area, where they breathed, and where their odours and the odours of their refuse and effusions collected and lingered.

Applying environmentalist reasoning after the fact, Ebenezer Beardsley explained high morbidity among George Washington's troops in 1776 as owing to the improper ventilation of their quarters.[41] Pringle, another military physician, wished to isolate the disease-conducive circumstances of military life. He turned his gaze upon the military hospital, an obvious site for the accumulation of corrupted air that transmits disease.[42] As correctives he advised the frequent movement of armies, improved privy facilities, and, most pertinently, the separation of patients in different hospitals according to their diseases.[43]

Behind these insights and inferences lay the physician's interest in pneumatic chemistry, and the persistent conviction, dating from Arbuthnot's 1733 essay, that research into the properties of the air would reveal its harmful components. The environmentalist thus followed the work of Priestley, Jean Sennebier, Jan Ingen-Housz, and others in pneumatic chemistry. This work showed that air of a certain quality cannot support life at all, which seemed to be proved by reports such as the story of the death of 123 out of 146 French soldiers imprisoned in le Trou noir – the black hole – in Bengal after being captured by British troops, and by experiments with animals given limited quantities of air (such as in small glass enclosures).[44] On the basis of such work the environmentalist concluded that there are degrees of mephitis, which the chemist will find ways to measure.

Pringle's ideas about the disease-conducive mechanism at work were influential both in Britain and on the European continent, and for that reason it is useful to consider them in more detail. These notions Pringle arrived at during service with the British army in Flanders in the War of Austrian Succession of the 1740s. Returning home after the war, Pringle continued to look for associations between noxious air and disease. On 1 February 1753 he reported a set of recent observations to members of the Royal Society in a paper entitled 'An Account of Several Persons Seized with the Gaol-Fever'.[45] In October 1750 the London court of alderman had appointed a commission to look into purifying the air of Newgate prison as a means of preventing jail fever, which most historical epidemiologists take to have been typhus. This step was prompted by the 'fatal instances [that] had occurred that year at the sessions held in the Old Bailey, when the lord mayor, two of the judges, and one of the aldermen upon the bench, with several other persons then present, were seized with a malignant fever, and died'.[46] The commission consulted Pringle, the leading theoretician of the noxious air–disease association, and Stephen Hales, a clergyman and physiologist best known at that time for his experiments with ventilators. Finding Newgate too small and crowded, Pringle and Hales recommended the reinstallation of ventilators, first used there in the 1740s. Municipal authorities would have less to fear when only healthy prisoners should be brought before them, and the ventilators would make the prison healthy.

Eighteenth-century physicians were not the first to detect an association between mephitic air and disease, but they did depart from convention in suggesting steps to be taken to redress the problem and avoid the diseases believed to arise in closed quarters. Ventilation, the periodic airing of these quarters (or, in more severe circumstances, the installation of mechanical equipment designed to force fresh air into the mephitic site), would disrupt the causal mechanism by dispelling the disease-laden air. An ally of ventilation was the chemical treatment: simmering vinegar; burning sulphur, tar, tobacco, even gunpowder; dispersing acids valued for their countervailing odour; or otherwise using chemical means to reduce, absorb, or dispel stench. All such measures promised to rid the habitations and buildings of the age of the harmful side of their paradoxical nature: buildings protect man from the elements but they also hold disease-causing forces within their walls.

Reinterment

Some stench-producing sites required other methods of treatment. To Noah Webster, for example, the refuse casually tossed into the streets of American towns and cities could not merely be flushed away but required periodic collection and disposal by burial or at sea. Finke claimed that the city of Berlin could reduce its annual mortality by 200 if its night soil were no longer thrown into the River Spree.

In addition to this generalised association between refuse and disease, the environmentalist detected a particularly pernicious source of urban mortality – the burial ground within the city, often inside churches. To Moheau and Daquin in France, to Devèze in Philadelphia, and to many physicians in other lands, these corpses should be reinterred outside the city, and future burials should occur only in sites detached from dense human habitation and contact.[47]

A century earlier William Petty, presumably writing tongue in cheek, had reassured his contemporaries that the historic population of the world had not been so great as to threaten the availability of space on Judgement Day.[48] The environmentalist worried, however, that the accumulation of corpses threatened the good health of the living population. As Iman Jacob van den Bosch reported, the mortality records of Amsterdam showed some 8 000 burials a year, yet the city had only seventeen churches available for these corpses.[49] The burial vaults within the churches were repeatedly being reopened. As a consequence visitors to the church, especially the faithful worshipping there, and even those who merely lived in the vicinity, were threatened with epidemic disease.

Elsewhere in the Dutch Netherlands Johan Diderik van Leeuwen, receiver-general of ordinary taxes in the old Roman town of Tiel, established a society to promote burials in special sites outside urban areas. At Tiel he laid out the Patriotische Kerkhof, the Patriotic Cemetery (Van Leeuwen had sided with the Patriot Party in the Dutch Revolution of 1787) with this inscription upon its gate:

> De menschenliefde door 't gezond verstand verlicht
> Heeft deez' begraafplaats tot een voorbeeld hier gesticht.
>
> (Humanity enlightened by common sense
> Has established here this cemetary as an example.)[50]

In Utrecht and elsewhere in the Republic a movement in favour at least of requiring future burials to occur outside the city, if not also to mandate the reinterment of corpses in existing sites, gained momentum in the second half of the eighteenth century.[51]

This campaign can be traced to the abbé Porée's 1744 examination of the dangers of interment within churches.[52] Later Henri Haguenot caught the imagination of eighteenth-century readers by reporting an account of multiple deaths from the consequences of opening a burial chamber in the parish church of Notre Dame in Montpellier. In adding the remains of a monastic brother to those of others in the common vaults of the church, the porter, Pierre Basalgette, was overcome. His associates went to his aid, but they too were convulsed as they descended into the chamber. Several of them died. Haguenot concluded that burials in common vaults, indeed within churches at all, are absolutely pernicious and should be prohibited.[53]

Warnings against the dangers of burial sites were already old in European medical literature before the abbé Porée turned his attention to this issue. Ramazzini could point both to Hippocrates and to the sixteenth-century humanist Giglio Giraldi as predecessors in their concern for corpse-bearers, an occupation especially vulnerable to disease because those who followed it breathed the mephitic air of burial vaults.[54] Early in the eighteenth century the controversialist Thomas Lewis attempted to prove that burial within churches had developed only during the medieval period, and therefore enjoyed no firm theological support.[55]

Such generalised concerns the environmentalist transformed into a specific campaign, to shift the dead away from the living. Historians of France, especially Richard Etlin, Madeleine Foisil, and Philippe Ariès, have developed the history of this campaign in that land.[56] I shall follow the campaign in other locations, especially the Dutch Netherlands, to show more of its breadth.

ENVIRONMENTAL ENGINEERING IMPLEMENTED

The beginnings of a broad effort aimed at disrupting the environment–disease association may be found in the 1740s and 1750s. The sources consulted for this book – the environmentalist literature of the eighteenth century, medical journals and journals containing epidemiological material, medical histories, and a variety of miscellaneous archival and printed sources encountered in research on this and other topics – reveal a multitude of specific instances of this campaign. No source that I have yet seen is devoted to it. My knowledge is thus piecemeal, and I cannot say whether these actions, which found their way into the records that I have consulted, represent a few, many, or a great volume of other measures of the same type. Let us, however, survey these actions in order to see what more specifically the environmentalists proposed to do to drain, lavate, ventilate, reinter, or otherwise elude pathogenic features of the environment, and what actions public authorities and public spirited citizens took toward the same end.

In Paris the street drainage system was improved in 1740 by walling in the outlet channels into which street gutters flowed.[57] That was followed in 1764 by introduction of a tax incentive (twenty years' freedom from all taxes and from the tithe levied by the church) to encourage drainage projects throughout France,[58] and later in the century by other urban sanitation improvements, including the use of suction pumps to empty cesspits.[59] Many British cities adopted Improvement Acts in the 1760s and thereafter, providing for street paving, widening, and cleansing, and for better sewage disposal.[60] These publicly and privately sponsored construction improvements, which followed a rebuilding of towns in brick, 'amounted to a significant modification of the urban environment'.[61] Prussian drainage projects designed to reduce contact with emanations from standing waters came to be cited elsewhere in Europe, for example in La Maillardière's study of drainage, as models suitable for emulation.[62] In the Dutch East Indian city of Batavia the governor general, Jacob Mossel, studying unusually heavy mortality in the periods 1733–8 and 1740–53, recommended a grand programme of swamp drainage and other measures to prevent the formation of pools of stagnant water.[63] During the remainder of the century these initial efforts were expanded upon. Drainage projects were executed in Scotland; in Portsmouth, England in 1769 and in its hinterland in 1793; in Hochberg, Baden; by Voltaire at his estate at Ferney; in numerous locales in the United States; and elsewhere.[64] In Italy Pope Pius VI revived an ancient programme of draining marshes in the vicinity of Rome, and Venetian authorities attempted to drain standing waters in certain parts of the Republic.

Nor was it only marshes and bogs that the environmentalists and their allies had in mind, but any situation in which standing water accumulated, collected natural, vegetable, or human refuse, and emitted a stench. Joseph II was thus persuaded to inaugurate a campaign to fill in moats and to raze needless fortifications whose high walls impeded air circulation.[65] These actions followed the promulgation in 1770 of a general public health law for the Empire, a law that established central government responsibility for public health. Here and there, including at the Bastille in Paris, moats were drained or allowed to dry up in order to reduce their mephitic exhalations (when the revolutionaries attacked the Bastille on 14 July 1789, they made their way over a moat that had long ago become dry). While doubting the effectiveness of French efforts at land clearance, André Bourde concludes that the 1764 edict to encourage drainage had an undoubted importance.[66] It renewed and expanded privileges for drainage measures and, together with improved techniques and a rise in land prices and rents, led to 'innumerable projects' organised by large and small private entrepreneurs.[67] The medicine of the environment also produced a literature on repairing the public health damages of floods, and on avoiding the ill consequences of drainage projects. This literature focused on lavation and ventilation.[68] These treatments of pathogenic sites in the environment thus overlapped.

Are these merely the annals of environmentalism? For the moment nothing else will suffice, for it remains necessary to show the breadth of these projects. Let us notice also the campaign in Switzerland led by the cleric and demographer Jean-Louis Muret. And let us notice that similar campaigns were mounted during the second half of the eighteenth century by the Vicomte de La Maillardière in France, by Richard Price and Joseph Priestley in Britain, first by Cadwallader Colden (in the 1740s) and later by others in the United States.[69] Indeed European proponents saw one of the most persuasive proofs of the public health efficacy of drainage in the American example, which combined drainage with deforestation. Most of Europe was already deforested. What remained to be done was to drain, thus to complete the dyad which to Europeans seemed to have played such an important role in rapid American population growth in the eighteenth century.[70] American experience with growth played an important part in informing Europeans about maximum possible rates of demographic expansion; to the populationists it described the optimum.[71]

To Americans the dyad of drainage and deforestation seemed responsible for a downward shift in mortality to a point at which the New World was no longer conspicuously less healthy than the Old. Early colonists in North America attributed heavy mortality to thick forests harbouring disease-causing forces, and its decline to forest clearance.[72] In time they came to discern a seasoning process, which most physicians explained in terms of adjustment to the rigours of the American climate, its excesses in heat, in moisture, and in violent changes in these and other phenomena. Environmentalist theory offered a remedy for the milieu that took such a toll before its new inhabitants became seasoned: deforestation would, as Lining explained, alter the climate.[73] In the 1780s Benjamin Rush urged the general expansion of cultivation into areas made up of forests as well as swamps as a means of moderating climatic extremes. It was his conviction that the differences between Europe and the United States in temperature and humidity extremes were already disappearing, which he inferred from observations in the state of Pennsylvania.[74] Rush's 1786 article, published in the *Transactions of the American Philosophical Society*, distinguished between deforestation in the vicinity of mill ponds, which was harmful because it allowed the free passage of marsh effluvia, and clearance with cultivation, which he found helpful. In the United States fevers had declined with cultivation except near mill ponds. Thus 'the Increase of Bilious and Intermitting Fevers in Pennsylvania' Rush attributed to a general increase in the number of mill ponds (and sites of standing waters), deforestation in their neighbourhoods, and the variable quantity of rainfall in recent years.

As a measure of improvement, drainage had the advantage of promising both economic and public health returns. The swamp thus treated would become an initially rich field, adding (for a few years at least) more to national output than a quantity in proportion to its size. Hence governments interested themselves in these measures, encouraging private drainage projects – such as France did with tax incentives – or by direct funding. The other leading measures for correcting pathogenic sites within the environment did not all have this same appeal. Lavation was described by its proponents as a measure that would merely improve public health. But the ventilation of urban space (in the form of street widening) served economic ends by allowing larger and heavier commercial traffic. And the transfer of cemeteries outside the city offered profitable opportunities for urban redevelopment.[75] Let us not underestimate the appeal to the inhabitants of a city or a region of the promise that certain measures, once undertaken, will diminish mortality. But let us recognise also the abstract quality of the promise. Lives will be saved, the environmentalists promised. But whose? How is anyone whose life has been saved to know that? The victims of a failure to act may be clearly known; the beneficiaries of action cannot. These economic motives thus provided the powerful incentive needed to transform idealism into action.

Lavation found its strongest adherents among those who would divert rivers and streams in order to flush refuse from city streets, and who would otherwise assure the cleansing of the city. In Philadelphia, Colden recommended diversion projects to flush the city's streets; in Amsterdam, Antony Grave explained the value of a more rapid circulation of water in the city's canals, into which most of the city's waste passed, and showed how to speed up circulation; in Paris, Claude Planche, 'entrepreneur in all types of projects related to wells', endorsed one Durozer's invention to prevent the seepage of foul water into wells; and in Montpellier the chemist Chaptal de Chanteloup urged that the water in cisterns be agitated in order to keep insects from establishing themselves in it.[76] The inattentiveness of urban historians to such issues as this makes it especially difficult to discover how widespread projects of lavation were, and whether those recommended were introduced or maintained.

Ventilation, in contrast, is known to have come into vogue in the 1740s and 1750s, and to have retained its appeal through the end of the century. When we left ventilation in the first part of this chapter, John Pringle and Stephen Hales had recommended the installation of ventilators in Newgate prison as a way of protecting judicial authorities from the risks of contact with diseased criminals. Ventilation devices were installed in some prison wards in June, 1752, and in July Pringle and Hales visited Newgate again. They found these wards 'much less offensive than the rest'.[77] Interviewing some prisoners, they learned that at first sickliness had increased, which Pringle attributed to the initial action of the first ventilator in drawing foul air from a large area through the ward first served. Subsequently, as the prisoners agreed, general healthiness had improved. Pringle and Hales were confident that these preliminary findings justified ventilation of all wards.

The precise grounds for this optimism Pringle chose to illustrate by citing the case of seven of eleven workmen among the installers taken ill during their labours.[78] In 1633 a group of Parisian physicians, asked to explain the deaths of five labourers who had just opened a sewer, attributed them to the pernicious gaze of a basilisk.[79] Pringle faced a similar problem, not the immediate death of any labourer but rather several cases of apparently the same malady that befell members of the labouring crew and their families. He found a solution in their mutual exposure to foul air. For example, Clayton Hand came down with a continued fever which, upon interviewing him, Pringle supposed to be owing to Hand's having opened a shaft closed for several years and breathed in the stench within. And when the family of another worker, Thomas Wilmot, came down with the same disease as Wilmot, Pringle attributed this to Wilmot's 'remarkably offensive' breath, sweat, and excrement. The foul air that killed Wilmot was transmitted by these means to his family, whose members became sick but did not die.[80] Such arguments sustained the case for installing ventilators in a variety of sites.

The great inventor of ventilation devices in Pringle's day was

Stephen Hales,[81] who read a paper on his mechanisms before the Royal Society in 1741. In the original form, Hales' machine was a hand-operated bellows intended to rid naval vessels of foul air, thus to prevent epidemics. Later he introduced windmill-operated devices, which were installed in Newgate prison, with the windmill situated on the roof, and on naval vessels. Hales' case for the public health benefits of ventilation construed these devices to be antiseptic, ridding closed areas of disease-causing vapours and cooling and sweetening the air. Their effectiveness he sought to demonstrate by a series of before-and-after comparisons of unhealthy sites transformed. In the London Small-Pox and Inoculation Hospital, for instance, the introduction of ventilators led to a third fewer deaths.[82] Some environmentalists even argued that Captain Cook's crew in the famous 1772–5 voyage had escaped scurvy because of ventilation and sanitation improvements rather than because of their consumption of citrus fruit.[83]

Among the most urgent arguments for ventilation may be found in the *Encyclopédie* and the *Journal encyclopédique*. In the first of these the authors Jaucourt and Formey endorsed Hales' devices and argued that they considered the utility of measures to provide air circulation in closed quarters as proven.[84] The *Journal encyclopédique* reported in 1762 that a ventilation mechanism had been installed in the House of Commons (J. T. Desaguliers' centrifugal bellows, in 1735), thereby summoning up in medicine the example of British superiority, which in the hands of people like Voltaire was so forceful an argument for reforms in French political practice. The reputed success of the House of Commons ventilator came repeatedly to be cited in France in proposals urging that similar mechanisms be installed in French buildings. Hales' hand-powered bellows, or the rival devices of Samuel Sutton, already introduced into a number of British naval vessels and hospitals, were installed on French merchant ships and, beginning in 1753, on French slavers. French naval authorities adopted a device invented by the Swede, Martin Triewald, which the Swedish navy had used first in its blockade of St Petersburg in 1741.[85] The British navy also used wind-sails and canvas tubes leading into crews' quarters, but their utility was more limited.[86] In 1774, inspired by the prison reformer John Howard, Parliament adopted legislation providing for the lavation and ventilation of prisons as well as separate quarters for diseased prisoners.[87] French hospitals began to duplicate these measures toward the end of century, initiating what emerged as a major nineteenth-century movement in the reform of hospital architecture that produced the pavilion style.[88] In Philadelphia, Ebenezer Robertson presented the American Philosophical Society with his model of a ventilation machine in 1793.[89]

Hales' devices, among the most widely used ventilators in eighteenth-century prisons, hospitals, and ships, and promoted enthusiastically by their inventor, proved difficult to keep in operation. The bellows required labourers to work them. At Newgate the use of a windmill for power was intended to overcome this problem, but its operation was sporadic until 1767, when the old prison was demolished. In the British navy a 1756 order provided for the installation of Hales' devices on all ships, but the extent to which the order was executed is uncertain.[90] Surveying hygienic conditions in British prisons and hospitals at the turn of the century, John Mason Good found a general improvement.[91] But he failed to undertake any systematic comparison. James Lind, one of the earliest proponents of the installation of ventilators on ships and in prisons, later came to the view that this measure had not in itself been sufficient. Infections had continued to occur.[92] The sources do not provide an account of unambiguous progress in the use of devices that would force air to circulate. Instead, they tell a story of increasingly widespread but probably in some cases still sporadic use of both old and new ventilation devices.

The campaign to transfer human remains away from contact with the living I have referred to under the heading 'reinterment'. Strictly speaking it was a campaign of interment and reinterment, for many environmentalists recommended the interment of wastes and the reinterment of corpses. It is especially the second action that had a large success in the eighteenth century. In 1775 Prussia ordered that in future burials should occur only outside towns and cities, a measure duplicated in other German states, Sweden, Modena, and elsewhere in following years.[93] In the Dutch Netherlands, Van Leeuwen's society, while meeting resistance from conservative forces within the Dutch Reformed Church, promoted the establishment of rural cemeteries.[94] At Tiel the rector of the Latin School, Ernst

Ephraim van Bergen, was the first person to be buried at the new site. His epitaph read, in part:

> His virtue and wisdom were too great
> That he should do harm after his death.

Burial inside churches was prohibited in the Netherlands by the new revolutionary government of 1795, reauthorised by William I in 1813, and finally forbidden in 1829.[95]

French environmentalists sought not merely to suspend new burials within churches but also to reinter the accumulated remains of centuries elsewhere. In Flanders and Artois the intendant Calonne ordered the exhumation and reinterment of cadavers that had been buried in the Church of Saint Eloi in Dunkirk since 1452. He wished merely to have the interior of the church rebuilt, but the experience of the surgeon he appointed (Hecquet) and of others involved in the project led to the publication of reports on it. Those explained what measures to take to protect public health while executing such projects.[96] In Paris later in the 1780s the Société royale de médecine sought to rid the city of one of its greatest centres of infection by reintering the corpses at the Church of the Holy Innocents. (The remains, in '11 898 cartloads by day, 3 475 carriages at night, 1 000 cartloads of bones', were transferred to catacombs, where they are still on view.)[97] In 1799 the suggestion was made that the department of the Seine create a *champ de repos* outside the city walls, in Montmartre.[98] Such a measure had been proposed for Paris as early as 1763, when the Parlement of Paris ordered that burial sites within the city be closed, to be replaced by eight large cemeteries outside Paris. A daily train of wagons was to collect corpses and transport them to the cemeteries. The order was not executed, 'probably because of its radicalism'.[99] The famous cemetery Père-Lachaise was not built until 1807. But the movement to transfer burials outside Paris began earlier.[100]

In *The Hour of Our Death*, Philippe Ariès links the shifting of old remains and the interment of the dead outside the city to profound changes in attitudes toward death in the Christian West.[101] In the eighteenth century, he argues, there arose a strong desire among the living to detach themselves from the dead, a desire that found expression in the relocation of burial sites and the creation of the cemetery as we now know it. The notion that the dead posed a threat to public health was, in this view, presumably a mere sign of a deeper shift in attitude. Ariès is persuaded that, until the eighteenth century, Latin Christendom was indifferent to the proximity of the dead buried close to the surface, to 'the daily presence of the living among the dead'.[102]

In the medical sources, I find a different emphasis. They reveal a shift in attitudes led by public health arguments, by the proposition that living amongst the dead is a cause of unnecessary mortality and morbidity. When the physician proposed to move the cemetery away from the church, to move the interred away from the holy relics of the church, and to reinter remains already within the church, he encountered resistance from the church and the populace. Only slowly, and by merging the public health campaign with the general Enlightenment effort to improve – to ameliorate discord between man and nature – did the physician find a way to persuade public and religious authorities to act. The case of Van Leeuwen and the Patriotic Cemetery at Tiel is telling. The environmentalist effort to detach the living from the dead preceded a change in popular attitudes, and helped cause it.

The movement to shift the site of burial outside the town and city emerged in the second half of the eighteenth century on the European continent. It was not a movement limited to countries where Roman Catholicism was the dominant religion, for burials within churches had continued in some countries after the Reformation. But it was not, alone among these improvements, general in Europe and North America. In neither Britain nor North America were significant numbers of people ever buried within churches, or in the shallow burial yards sometimes encountered on the European continent. Only local notables and high church officials were buried within English churches, and there ancient towns traced cemeteries outside the city to Roman times.

CONCLUSION

In the eighteenth century arose the expectation that pathogenic features of the environment might be modified, thereby to reduce disease and deaths. The enviromentalists had a general sense of the harmful nature of some environmental forces, and especially of as yet still largely unidentified complexes of forces. They had also one specific idea – that stench is an unambiguous sign of the pathogen. If therefore the causal nexus remained unclear, the evidence of its existence could not be doubted. Thus fell to the environmentalist the task of devising a strategy of avoidance and prevention. Drainage, lavation, ventilation, and interment and reinterment constituted the principal measures of environmental modification. Their application would disrupt the environment–disease association.

Let us recognise here not the new attitude toward death, which Ariès detects, but a new sensitivity to scent. Europeans had not discovered their own odours. But they had discovered the odours of their milieu and formed a distaste for them. The rich historiography of the late twentieth century has produced its student of odour. Alain Corbin detects in the eighteenth century a mutation in human sensibility toward odour.[103] Here is another merger of philosophy and medicine, for the mutation finds its origin in the writings of Locke and Condillac on sensory perception. Since the odours of the age were not new, the interesting question is – why this sudden sensitivity to them? Perhaps the answer arises from nothing more than the development of the notion that the unpleasant might be avoided, that it is possible for man to modify nature. If the *philosophes* were often scornful of the medicine of the individual, there is a large overlap between their agenda for the reform of man and nature, and the campaign of the environmentalists.

Let us notice also that environmental action occurred at three levels: central government, local and town government, and private initiative. The story of increasingly effective public and private action in the arena of 'social precautions' – to use a phrase provided by Eric Jones – is a story usually told around the rising efficacy of measures against the plague. It is a study that Jones prefers to recount in terms of the declining general incidence of disasters in the West from the sixteenth century onward, and the rising effectiveness of the state in managing or eluding disasters – epidemics, famines, and natural catastrophes.[104] The history of environmental action is a part of this still larger story, for it is specific to the period from the 1740s on, when, under public and private sponsorship, there emerged a generalised attack on epidemic disease in place of a specialised attack on the plague. This attack was fostered and made aggressive by coinciding with the humanitarianism of the eighteenth century, according to which thinkers in all areas of human curiosity imagined that it is possible to improve the lot of man.

6 Medical Effects of Environmental Engineering

> the most effectual means
> of guarding against . . .
> diseases.[1]
>
> Bisset

Did the medicine of the environment influence health? Specifically, did it diminish morbidity and mortality, as its practitioners wished it to do? The eighteenth-century sources consulted for this book do not provide a conclusive answer to these questions. They focus on the theory of the medicine of the environment, on the measures proposed by the environmentalists, and on measures implemented. They do not always discuss untreated sites, and they do not furnish satisfactorily detailed evidence about treated sites.

The environmentalists themselves had no doubts. They regarded their efforts to diminish morbidity and mortality as successful, and saw mankind standing on the eve of great victories over epidemic disease. William White thus examined the bills of mortality and found public health in York to have improved between 1728–35 and 1770–6, which he attributed to interim improvements: street widening and cleaning, and the construction of a drainage system.[2] Others based their arguments about the efficacy of environmental engineering on more conventional claims. Frank cited classical sources reporting improved public health after the implementation of measures such as he recommended in his general program of medical police.[3] And more generally the environmentalists accepted the logic of their own case: there is an association of influence or causation between the environment and disease; treatment of the environment will disrupt it.

These sources of confidence will not be counted persuasive

today. But the historical evidence on mortality in eighteenth-century Europe reveals a decided downward trend, evident especially in the European core, in Western Europe and Britain.[4] In cities and in the countryside, mortality rates declined. Their decline would continue in the nineteenth century. Morbidity, in contrast, remains a great unknown. Presumably the regression of mortality signals a coincidental regression of morbidity but, in the absence of direct evidence, all assumptions about morbidity remain speculative.

The decline in mortality can be attributed to a decline in infectious diseases, and specifically in the frequency and severity of epidemics, but different authorities have approached explanations of this phenomenon in different ways. Thomas McKeown assigns most of the nineteenth-century decline in infectious diseases to a fall in mortality from air-borne infections (such as tuberculosis and smallpox) rather than water- and food-borne diseases (such as cholera, which first appeared in Europe as an epidemic in the nineteenth century) or insect-borne diseases.[5] In contrast, Stephen Kunitz speculates about an increase in population density which may have converted crowd diseases into more benign childhood diseases.[6]

Much of the attention on infection has been directed toward plague. Thus McKeown's relegation of insect-borne diseases to a role of little importance in the mortality reduction is based chiefly on an attempt to disassociate the earlier decline in plague mortality, a seventeenth-century phenomenon, from the reduction in mortality since the eighteenth century. To be specific, McKeown combines diseases also transmitted by insects with food- and water-borne diseases, overlooks the extended effects of malaria as a debilitating disease, underestimates the effects of a decline in other insect-borne diseases, and leaves the impression that the overall mortality decline was concentrated in diseases (tuberculosis and smallpox) known not to have diminished in incidence on the continent before the nineteenth century.[7] While it is appropriate to doubt the role of vector-borne plague and water-borne cholera in the eighteenth-century decline in mortality, it is premature to conclude that other insect- or food- and water-borne diseases did not experience a change in incidence during the eighteenth century.

This chapter will search the actions of the environmentalists for measures that may have contributed to the eighteenth-century decline in mortality rates. Of course this search involves a paradox. The environmentalists wished to treat the milieu in order to avoid or diminish human contact with agents, forces, and factors now known not to be direct causes of disease. Specifically, they construed the causes of disease in terms of non-living forces and factors and, although corpuscular theorists, thereby failed to guess the presence of disease-causing microorganisms. And they fostered a theory of disease communication of which some elements – such as particles of disease-causing matter carried in the air – seem very close to today's ideas, and others – such as stench as a disease agent – seem decidedly anachronistic. The issue here, however, is not whether the environmentalists came a step (or several steps) closer to identifying the actual causes of disease or the vectors that often transmit disease. The issue is whether the measures they proposed to take to treat the pathogenic environment actually disrupted environments in which disease-causing microorganisms, and the living vectors of disease transmission, thrived. Did the environmentalists, more unwittingly than wittingly, treat the primary causes of disease, of which bacteria and infectious material, and the vectors that sometimes transmit them, are secondary causes?

EIGHTEENTH-CENTURY MORTALITY

At the beginning of the century, historical demographers now estimate, Europe's population totalled some 110 million. By 1750 it had risen to some 140 million, and by 1800 to perhaps 187 million.[8] Thus began a pattern of growth that carried the population of that continent to some 690 million in 1980. The great issues in the eighteenth-century movement of the European population are fertility and mortality. Migration can be an important matter, but the population increase does not seem to have been influenced significantly by sometimes quite large internal migrations,[9] and it occurred in spite of a net outflow of people, chiefly in the form of emigration to the New World. Here attention falls on mortality, the decline of which seems to have been the principal source of population growth on the European continent, and an important but perhaps secondary contributor to growth in England.[10]

If the question is clear, the answer is not. Historians have considered many possible explanations for the decline in mortality, usually thinking in terms of the applicability of a specific force to a specific region or country. Most of these explanations can be rejected because they cannot explain a large enough part of the observed decline, or because they were not sufficiently widespread to explain a phenomenon of population growth that itself transcended national boundaries.

Medical science has of course figured in this search for an explanation. Earlier historians tended to accept the eighteenth-century physicians' own claims about the efficacy of medicine, but in an often-cited 1955 essay Thomas McKeown and R. G. Brown considered these claims and rejected them.[11] The eighteenth-century medicine of the individual – specifically surgery, midwifery, and medicines – does not appear to have significantly reduced the mortality rate. More recently, Peter Razzell has argued that smallpox inoculation (which was introduced in England in the 1720s) may explain the English growth of the eighteenth century.[12] But if inoculation had such a large impact in England, which other authorities have doubted,[13] it clearly did not have the same effect elsewhere, where it was introduced later and less systematically.[14]

Attention has focused also on improvements in nutrition, and specifically on greater agricultural output in combination with more regular and efficient distribution of basic food items.[15] The inference that improved nutrition was a leading cause of mortality decline is strong in the demographic literature, and is a particularly noteworthy feature of McKeown's attempt to explain the decline in infectious disease in England. But it is poorly substantiated by evidence about agricultural output and about improvements in transportation and food supply administration. Some areas (for example, England) may have experienced increased *per capita* output in the eighteenth century.[16] For others, however, output is believed merely to have kept pace with population growth (France), or to have diminished while the population grew (Eastern Europe). In Germany agricultural output exceeded population growth, but in a labour intensive manner detrimental to net nutrition.[17] Even in England, where *per capita* income is believed to have grown, most estimates indicate that the growth rate of grain yields was not as high as that of population. Furthermore, population growth was paralleled by increasing food prices, leaving open the question of whether higher incomes meant better nutrition.

Considering the issue of the administrative management of food supplies by comparing price disparities among different markets, Louise Tilly found that in France the largest shift toward similar prices occurred before the middle of the seventeenth century – that is, before the late seventeenth- or early eighteenth-century disappearance of the classic subsistence crisis that figures so prominently in French studies of price and population history.[18] Elsewhere studies of market integration, and therefore of changes in efficiency of foodstuff distribution, have as yet made little headway.

Another problem with the nutrition hypothesis arises from its assumption that infectious disease is necessarily related to poor nutrition. Many diseases believed to have been common causes of death – plague, malaria, smallpox, and typhoid – are not significantly related to nutrition in onset or fatality rate, and others – influenza, typhus, and probably tuberculosis – have an equivocal relationship.[19] Biochemical evidence suggests that 'undernutrition does not make the human body prone to more severe or more frequent infection', and Ann Carmichael points up a 'synergism between disease and disease rather than between nutritional status and disease'.[20] Considering the case of eighteenth-century England, it seems especially unlikely that poor nutrition will have been as significant as McKeown implies in a society whose *per capita* income was either the highest or second highest in the world, and two or three times higher than that in some less developed twentieth-century economies, such as India and Nigeria in the 1960s.[21]

Some attention has also been given 'a diminution of the severity, frequency and ubiquity of [mortality] crises', which M. W. Flinn assigns to the second half of the seventeenth century.[22] Famine crises became less frequent in England after 1597, in France after the 1690s, and in other places at other times. But this shift may be found in this period only in Western Europe. There, Flinn believes, crises were diffused. The poor no longer died from disease induced by inadequate nourishment, but remained poorly nourished and susceptible to epidemics.[23] Later, in the eighteenth century, mortality from infectious diseases diminished. 'Something was done, some actions were taken, which prevented the epidemics from exacting such a high toll'.[24] This hypothesis also suffers from the necessary link it draws between famine and epidemic disease. But it acknowledges a long-continuing story of mortality decline, one in which different forces may have to be cited to explain different phases. Eric Jones has identified one factor as 'deliberate attempts by the nation-states of pre-industrial times to "manage" disasters'.[25] Central governments reduced the effects of harvest failures by storing larger quantities of grain. Most of Jones' case rests on the use of quarantines in epidemics and epizootics, however, and it is difficult to evaluate the effectiveness of quarantines in an age in which wealthier people, often on their physician's advice, fled at the first signs of an epidemic, quarantine or not.

Another factor of possible influence is a secular warming trend, which assisted output or moderated the mortality extremes associated with heat and cold. But of climatic melioration, recent evidence suggests that only marginal areas of Europe are likely to have been much affected.[26]

The last category of hypotheses, the one to which the hypothesis formulated here belongs, is grouped around the idea of a changing pattern of infectious disease. Many commentators mention (but do not develop) the possibility of changes in the virulence of microorganisms, although McKeown specifically rejects a decline in virulence as a general explanation for the decline in mortality.[27] It is difficult to find evidence that will allow a test of this possibility, or to establish what form any changes in virulence may have taken. In the eighteenth century any changes in the biological nature of microorganisms are unlikely to have been influenced by human actions – e.g., by drugs in the way that such mutations today are associated with antibiotics – so that this hypothesis raises the uncomfortable issue of fortuity. It is true also that the pattern of declining mortality does not appear to have followed trade routes, such as those linking the Baltic to Britain and the Dutch Republic, and it is along such routes that one should expect mutant microorganisms to have been dispersed. Furthermore, it is implausible to suppose that mutations will, in large numbers, be skewed only toward diminished virulence. In biological theory mutations should be expected to be randomly distributed along a virulence curve. If the virulence hypothesis is meant to refer to resistance to disease, then it begs the question, for the issue then is what events may have heightened popular resistance to disease.

Shifting the point of attention, Kunitz suggests the hypothesis of a change in the biology of microorganisms, by which he means improved human control over disease-causing events (wars) and over disease transmission, specifically of the plague. This is suggested to have occurred together with a change in the age-specific incidence of certain infectious diseases (louse-borne typhus, tuberculosis, smallpox, and measles), which ceased to be crowd diseases and became more benign childhood diseases.[28] This putative change he associates with increased population density, which diminished isolation from diseases. Kunitz does not raise the possibility of human action upon disease itself. This form of the hypothesis, more a speculation than an hypothesis, also has shortcomings. Population densities varied quite substantially across Europe, and are not known to have varied in a pattern consonant with the regression of mortality, as would be expected from Kunitz' hypothesis. The eighteenth-century trend of population in England was upward, but in the nearby Dutch Republic (another densely settled region) the trend was nearly stable, and urbanisation may have diminished. Furthermore, this idea uses population growth itself to explain population growth, leaving moot the initiation of the event.

Each of these hypotheses possesses both strengths and weaknesses, and each proceeds along the difficult path of reasoning from effect. Only the event itself is identified, leaving the historian to search for a cause. The hypothesis that environmental changes reduced the incidence of epidemic disease shares this characteristic. But it has the advantage of calling attention to a variety of measures undertaken across Europe in the eighteenth century toward the specific goal of lessening the number and impact of epidemic diseases.

When McKeown and Brown considered the possibility of a medical explanation for the eighteenth-century rise of population, they specifically rejected an explanation based on therapies for treating the patient. They considered and neither accepted nor rejected an explanation drawing on public health reforms: 'Improvements in the environment are . . . regarded as intrinsically the most acceptable explanation of the decline in mortality in the late eighteenth and nineteenth centuries'.[29] But they did not inquire whether extensive modifications of the English environment occurred, and turned their attention away from environmental engineering as discussed here and toward the issue of agricultural improvements that may have augmented food production.[30] Although McKeown and Brown left open the possibility of a public health explanation, most authorities have either ignored or rejected this possibility. Jacques Dupâquier, considering the eighteenth-century decline of mortality in France, argues that public health reforms cannot have been responsible. They were limited to towns, which included only 18 – 20 per cent of the total population.[31]

This rejection is premature. About public health too little has been done to investigate or test the demographic ramifications of specific measures. In this book we have considered a wide variety of improvements suggested by the environmentalists. Some of these have been identified in the literature, especially by McKeown and Brown. Others are new to historical demography (although not to the history of medicine). Some of these measures – lavation, ventilation, and reinterment especially – should be expected to have had their greatest impact on urban sites, or at least on densely populated quarters, such as the ship, the prison, and the hospital. Others – especially drainage – may be expected to have had their principal influence in the countryside. In any event, environmentalism was not exclusively an urban movement, although the environmentalists identified the town and city as an especially harmful site of pathogens. They recognised that mortality in towns and cities was higher than in the countryside, and therefore that gains in population from reducing urban mortality would be disproportionately large. It is thus appropriate to ask whether the medicine of the environment contributed to the regression of mortality. It is a question with precedent. Considering the grand medical *enquête* inaugurated in France in 1776, Jean Meyer has asked whether this provides a reason behind French demographic expansion in the latter years of the old regime.[32] Let us extend the question to cover those areas of the world where environmentalist measures were introduced, and those portions of the eighteenth century when such measures were common.

In a general study of the European demographic system in the early modern period, Flinn turned attention toward the possibility of an explanation for population growth based on improved 'welfare policies'.[33] In Flinn's judgement, it is necessary to look both at economic progress and at the 'primitive humanitarianism' of the eighteenth century, which in medicine revealed itself in efforts at disease avoidance more than in newly successful therapies. Another student of eighteenth-century death (rather than of mortality), John McManners, has joined this search by attributing the numerical expansion of mankind in eighteenth-century France in part to 'reforming [medical] administrators [who] established the main principles of public hygiene and social medicine as we know them'.[34]

It is in this construction that latitude may be found for a public health explanation for part of the eighteenth-century decline of mortality and morbidity (and, insofar as morbidity influences fertility, perhaps also for the increase of fertility). Flinn did not specify all the measures he had in mind under the rubric of 'welfare policies'. But it is clear that these include the environmental engineering steps discussed here. The inclusion has two features. It is, on one side, an affair of medicine and epidemiology. Physicians, persuaded that the environment is sometimes pathogenic, devised a set of treatments to avoid and prevent epidemic disease. It is, on the other side, a point of contact between medicine and the public spiritedness of the second half of the eighteenth century, between medicine and the reformist efforts of central and municipal governments, between medicine and Enlightenment humanitarianism in general. In seeking to modify nature and prevailing modes of human adaptation to nature to render it (and man's adaptation to it) less noxious, physicians found a host of allies.

The power of this revised and enlarged treatment of medicine and public health to explain the regression of mortality is also limited. Population growth can be discerned outside the temporal boundaries of the campaign to modify the environment. For example, the most recent research traces the beginning of French growth to the late seventeenth century,[35] to a time preceding any reasonable expectation that environmentalist measures significantly influenced growth. Where this putative effect seems to have been concentrated is in the 1740s onward.

What specifically may be expected from environmentalist action? Three measures – drainage, lavation, and ventilation – can be expected to have intruded upon ordinary contact between man and pathogens in the environment, and especially to have diminished human contact with some specific vectors transmitting disease.

DRAINAGE AND MALARIA

No one will doubt that the drainage of standing water can be an effective means to prevent malaria. To the eighteenth-century physician drainage removed a site at which environmental forces capable of causing disease came together, a site recognisable because of the higher mortality rate of nearby populations and because of its signs: odour and particulate matter in suspension in the air. To the twentieth-century epidemiologist and medical entomologist, standing water, especially small ponds and puddles, are breeding places for the mosquito species that act as vectors in transmitting this disease. (The malaria parasite was not discovered until 1880, and the role of the mosquito as vector was not proved until later still.) In Europe and North America malaria is usually transmitted by the *Anopheles* mosquito which, in the course of feeding, transfers plasmodium, the infectious matter, from an infected organism to a healthy organism. It is characterised by chills (ague), the recurrent appearance every three or four days of fever, spleen enlargement, and other symptoms. Hence certain descriptions of disease in seventeenth- and eighteenth-century mortality registers (especially ague and intermittent fevers) are usually taken to refer to malaria. For treatment eighteenth-century physicians came increasingly to recommend cinchona bark, which contains quinine. This is an effective drug in certain dosages for suppressing the clinical symptoms. No cure was known, and quinine dosages were not always given, or given in appropriate dosages.[36]

Eighteenth-century mortality records and medical literature provide evidence that diseases usually construed to have been malaria were common, but that they were not major causes of death. Malaria's case fatality rate is generally low except among children. In twentieth-century economically underdeveloped regions, this disease is often referred to as the great debilitator – as a common disease that robs the populace of part of its energy and increases susceptibility to other diseases. Today also it is not known by itself as a major killer.

Studying malaria eradication in Ceylon and British Guiana in the mid-twentieth century, Peter Newman found that 'where malaria is severely endemic, the eradication of the disease is bound to bring in its train very strong effects on the rate of population growth'.[37] This view rests on evidence which shows that 'endemic and even epidemic malaria, in its role as "the great debilitator", tends to reduce markedly the general healthiness and resistance to disease of the population at risk, and so to aggravate substantially the mortality effects of other diseases'.[38] Newman estimates all deaths caused by malaria to have been five times the number of deaths directly from malaria.[39] The indirect effects of malaria are thus believed, on the basis of twentieth-century evidence about endemic, epidemic, and severely epidemic malaria regions, to be much larger than the direct effects.

At some point since the seventeenth century malaria has been in regression across the world. Various measures, chief among them epidemiological surveillance, have reduced the incidence of this disease in North America where it was still common in some regions in the early nineteenth century, in Mediterranean Europe, and in Africa, Asia, and Latin America. This pattern of regression leads to the inference that malaria was at one time a disease of widespread incidence in much of the world, and that its comparative insignificance in nineteenth-century Europe is an indication of an earlier regression there. Dale Smith maintains that malaria was endemic throughout Europe in the eighteenth century.[40] But there is some doubt in the literature of historical epidemiology about the pre-nineteenth-century range of this disease, about its trend, and about the weight that should be assigned to several factors believed potentially responsible for the decline in malaria morbidity and mortality where such a decline is known to have occurred, and for the putative decline where such a trend is merely plausible.

Does the seventeenth- and eighteenth-century form of this disease appear, from the available evidence, to resemble closely the twentieth-century form? Recent investigations suggest significant variations in mortality among confirmed eigteenth-century malaria patients.[41] In the Dombes region of eighteenth-century France, for example, the inhabitants were recognisable because of their emaciation, indolence, swollen bellies, indifference, and other characteristics of long-term infection.[42] While the literature is rich in references to morbidity that is probably malarial, it is not rich in discussions of debilitation, and in particular it fails to enlighten about the unremarkable instances of long-term suffering from milder forms of this disease. How serious the problem of debility may have been in the eighteenth century remains unanswered. It is unlikely that old regime Europeans suffered quite the levels of debility identified in some twentieth-century regions of the world, where other and more virulent strains of the disease are known. But how much milder the European forms may have been is not known. At present, there are no grounds for refusing to apply evidence from twentieth-century investigations, as long as allowance is made for the likelihood of less virulent strains in eighteenth-century Europe than in twentieth-century tropical regions.

If there is an unanswered question about the historical nature and effect of the disease, there is also in the epidemiological literature a debate about the historic range of endemic malaria. Some authorities believe that its range in Europe was limited, although they do not always make clear whether the limited range reflects prior regression in areas where the disease had been prevalent or endemic, or whether it constitutes a more accurate statement about the range of territory in which malaria had ever been common.[43] In the language of the eighteenth century 'malaria' referred both to corrupt air and (less frequently) to a particular disease believed to be caused by such air. Linguistic ambiguity must thus be added to the variety of ailments designated as 'fever' as a problem complicating retrospective diagnoses. McKeown doubts that English marsh fever was plasmodium malaria and that temperatures in England were high enough for malaria to have been common,[44] but these doubts can certainly be set aside. One reason is that McKeown and some other authorities have overlooked entomological evidence about the twentieth-century distribution of appropriate *Anopheles* strains,[45] which is one way to estimate earlier distributions. Another reason is that numerous sources provide conclusive evidence that a disease believed to have been malaria was a major cause of illness and death in early modern Europe, at least as far north as the sixtieth degree of latitude. Bruce-Chwatt and de Zulueta show that malaria was common in both England and Scotland,[46] and Chambers holds that malaria was a major cause of death in pre-industrial England whose declining importance can be explained by drainage and other agricultural improvements.[47] Anning, working from a case book from 1781–4, reports that ague was far and away the most common diagnosis (28 per cent) among patients admitted to the Leeds General Infirmary, in north central England.[48] Some eighteenth-century British physicians described malaria (or diseases identifiable as malaria) as a serious problem,[49] and subsequently some epidemiologists (such as F. Bisset Hawkins, writing in 1829) cited drainage programmes for their contribution to reduced mortality. Indeed, Hawkins believed that drainage demonstrated man's capacity to accommodate himself to a less than optimally favourable climate, and considered it in a class with smallpox vaccination as a medical improvement.[50]

Other authorities acknowledge an earlier prevalence of malaria in middle and parts of northern Europe, but provide different estimates of the period of regression. McNeill suggests that in England the principal period of malaria regression came between 1650 and 1750. He attributes this to a spread of convertible husbandry and the growth of livestock herds (which provided a preferred feeding grounds for mosquitoes), but supplies no information about livestock populations.[51] As Bruce-Chwatt and de Zulueta notice, living in close proximity to stabled domestic animals may protect human populations.[52] Such a pattern had been common in seventeenth-century and earlier dwellings in low-lying regions, as a visitor to sites such as the Flemish historical park at Bokrijk, in Belgium, will discover by noticing that dwellings from that period (now relocated on higher ground) often placed humans in one side of a long house and animals in the other side. One might thus speculate about an increase in malaria incidence as house plans changed, and livestock were quartered in outbuildings.

Ackerknecht maintains that the regression of malaria came in the eighteenth and nineteenth centuries in Europe in general, and that it was owing to several factors working in harmony: drainage, larger cattle herds, ubanisation, and other changes.[53] In the view of Bruce-Chwatt and de Zulueta, however, the incidence of malaria in Europe increased during the seventeenth *and* eighteenth century before diminishing in the nineteenth, especially after 1850, as the result of human intervention, one form of which was epidemiological surveillance.[54] Hackett holds that endemic malaria peaked in Europe and North America around 1860.[55]

When the authorities disagree about so much, their disagreements spring simply from the lack of evidence. In this instance, they spring also, I believe, from a lack of knowledge about eighteenth-century drainage efforts. The arguments about malarial zones and periods of regression are usually based not on evidence about malaria but on the trend of other variables which are known, from subsequent experience, to have some significance in malaria aetiology. Knowing of the drainage campaign, we know therefore of grounds for suspecting an eighteenth-century regression. But the grounds will not be persuasive until we learn more about the actual incidence and range of malaria. In search of this additional information, let us shift our attention from the general to the specific case.

Mary Dobson examined mortality rates in marshy and non-marshy regions of England.[56] In the marshy areas of Essex and Kent, crude burial rates were exceptionally high in the sixteenth, seventeenth, and early eighteenth centuries because of the incidence of agues and fevers. After the early eighteenth century mortality diminished in 'an oscillating downward trend' that lasted until the mid-nineteenth century.[57] Did plasmodium malaria figure prominently as a cause of death, and why did mortality diminish? Dobson finds the evidence strongly suggestive of plasmodium malaria, pointing out also that an appropriate mosquito vector was (and still is) common in these regions. As to why mortality diminished, Dobson provides an extended list of factors that may have accounted for the decline, a list beginning with drainage and including larger livestock herds, better ventilated houses (which, with larger herds, contributed to a dissociation of man and mosquitoes), cinchona bark and quinine drugs, increased tolerance for the disease among inhabitants of the region, improved nutrition and general health, and perhaps also a change in the development of the relevant parasite. No single factor seems adequate to account for a regression evident in several areas at once, and so Dobson (unaware of the environmentalists' drainage campaign) proposes the hypothesis of different blends of these factors operating in different regions.[58]

Other scholars have also assigned drainage an interdependent rather than an independent role in the decline of malaria morbidity and mortality. But Dobson, accepting West's explanation for the decline of infant mortality in the Fenland parish of Wrangle after 1734, assigns drainage the role of a leading factor.[59]

Although beyond doubt effective, drainage is usually identified as the costliest (and thus the least practical) of the several techniques employed in malaria eradication in Europe in the campaign that began at the end of the Second World War and extended into the early 1970s.[60] Mid-twentieth-century governments allocate a far larger share of expenditures to social infrastructure improvements than did their eighteenth-century counterparts, which spent chiefly on wars and war debts.[61] But the drainage projects discussed in the environmentalist literature were not sponsored by central governments. They relied upon private initiative, and sometimes upon direct assistance from local governments or indirect aid from central governments (for example, in the form of tax incentives). Clearly old regime governments were capable of introducing and sustaining large hydraulic projects. The Dutch Netherlands had created and maintained an intricate hydraulic network designed to reclaim agricultural land, and stood in Europe as a model of hydraulic engineering and as a training ground for engineers. The Netherlands was not declared free of residual malaria endemicity until 1970, the same year as Italy.[62] Of course, malaria eradication occurs in two (or more) stages. In one, the goal is to reduce sharply the general incidence of the disease by bringing the mosquito population below the critical level of vector density necessary to make malaria a serious threat.[63] In the other, the goal is to eradicate all cases arising from domestic sources. The former is far more productive in terms of reduced morbidity and mortality, and it is the chronological location of this stage which is so important in assessing the role of malaria in early modern European mortality and morbidity.

Nevertheless it is appropriate to be suspicious about the extent to which eighteenth-century drainage projects may have been sustained in the long run. Dobson's finding of 'an oscillating downward trend' is suggestive of drainage efforts that, in the medium run, waxed and waned in their effects. Such a scheme is in accordance with what we know about eighteenth-century administrative efforts – it was an age in which people dreamed more grandly than they executed their many projects for improving life. This pattern also agrees with the expectation that innovation often met popular resistance. We have encountered that in the movement to reinter corpses buried within churches. Archival sources reveal it also in the drainage movement.

In the early 1770s the French controller general was called on to intervene in a dispute threatening violence in the parish of Annoeullin in Flanders where peasant opposition to drainage was especially intense.[64] Peat diggers in the area, digging fuel, had transformed formerly productive land into marshes.

Community leaders petitioned the intendant of Flanders and Artois for permission to clear and drain the marshes, but troops sent to assist in that were greeted with 'mutinerie et rébellion', as the intendant reported. Unable to decide between the interests of the propertied inhabitants of Annoeullin and the impoverished peat diggers, the intendant referred the dispute to the controller general.[65]

Elsewhere in late old regime France administrative sources indicate that drainage projects pitted those who would retain common rights to village land against those who would divide the commons and who wished to take advantage of royal edicts favouring clearance and drainage in order to force division.[66] In many communities, these disputes lasted for years and were brought to a conclusion only by the French Revolution, which not so much resolved them as disrupted the process of record keeping.

What do we know, and what do we need to know, about drainage and malaria? Dobson provides a case study in which drainage and other public health and social improvements may plausibly be cited as the causes behind the decline of mortality in some regions of England. Applying wisdom from modern experience to the analysis of historical instances, Dobson also discusses in a reasonable manner the extended effects of high malarial morbidity: diminished resistance to other diseases, including typhoid and influenza; added complications to other diseases; and chronic ill health and early death among malaria sufferers.[67] The eighteenth-century medical literature establishes the wide prevalence of diagnoses – chiefly ague and intermittent fever, but also fevers in general where no more detail is given – of which some at least seem to have been malaria and the undifferentiated fevers common in areas of endemic malaria. This literature pushes the eighteenth-century range of this disease far beyond its limits in twentieth-century Europe, and reminds us of anecdotal evidence about the importance of such fevers as causes of death among workmen building Louis XIV's palace at Versailles, and Peter the Great's city, St Petersburg. Environmentalist sources establish, moreover, that drainage was settled upon as an effective treatment of prevention for diseases among people living in the vicinity of standing water, especially swamps. And these same sources reveal that drainage projects were mounted in many locales during the 1740s, the 1750s, and succeeding decades. Drainage projects continued also to be undertaken in order to add arable land, and these unrelated projects (which gathered momentum with population growth itself and the rising demand for food) should also have contributed to a malaria regression associated with drainage.

The things we do not know are also numerous. What was the range of malaria in eighteenth-century Europe? How severe was endemicity in Europe in general, and in specific regions? How serious was malaria as a disease that had debilitating effects, and as a disease diminishing resistance to or complicating other ailments? How widespread was drainage? These questions simply cannot be answered conclusively from the evidence now available. To answer them requires more case studies of the type executed by Dobson – case studies which, if they tell the same story, will add to the assurance with which conclusions may be drawn.

In the meantime, the weight of the evidence argues both the importance of malaria as a disease and a cause of death in the seventeenth century (especially among children) and its much reduced significance by the mid- to late-nineteenth century. Certainly the range of the mosquito vector was wider than some authorities have acknowledged, and included (and still includes) England, a large portion of Scandinavia, and most of the rest of the continent. The appropriate strains do not remain active throughout the year in Europe, but overwinter and resume activity wherever the mean summer isotherm is at least 60°F. Drainage efforts coincided with the regression of malaria, although they may not have been solely responsible for the reduction of the mosquito population below the level necessary to preserve malaria as a major endemic disease. Mosquito control efforts continued to the middle of the twentieth century in areas of especially stubborn malaria endemicity, for example in parts of the Netherlands and Italy.

VENTILATION AND LAVATION

Stench and the effluvia of man and nature figured in an important way in the theory of disease propagation developed by the medicine of the environment, and therefore the avoidance of these things came to be seen as another means of reducing the incidence of epidemic disease. To avoid mephitis the environmentalist recommended many therapies, but all of them fall into two categories. In one the physician proposed to treat the open environment – by lavation, interment, drainage, or another technique. In the other the physician proposed to treat closed quarters – which were to be ventilated and sometimes also to be lavated or treated with an 'antiseptic' measure, such as simmering vinegar to force it to vaporise or by burning large sulphur matches. By either method stench (and thereby the source of disease) would be removed or covered up, or replaced by a 'healthy' odour. Dobson suggests that ventilation made human quarters less attractive to mosquitoes, who were thus encouraged 'to seek resting places amongst the animals'.[68] For the moment, however, we are concerned not with the effects of ventilation or the eighteenth-century form of antisepsis upon living vectors of disease, but the effects of these measures on air-borne contagion.

These things were to be done in the human dwelling, the church and every structure where people gathered – the prison, the ship, and the hospital. Let us explore what was done in the last of these, where disease lived. In the old regime the hospital provided care for the sick as well as for the disabled, the old, and the wretched. What the environmentalists proposed to do to improve these institutions ran parallel to a reform programme advanced by humanitarians concerned less with disease than with relieving misery.

In the middle of the century the hospital had the reputation of being a centre of disease and death. The humanitarians proposed to close the worse of these institutions, such as the Parisian hôtel-dieu, the 'tombeau du Peuple',[69] and to replace it with a system of domiciliary care and small neighbourhood hospices. The environmentalists proposed rather that existing institutions be reformed, enlarged, and made more numerous.[70] Between the 1780s and 1805, as the statistician Jacques Peuchet reported, more than 700 hospitals and 100 small infirmaries were built in France, providing substantial opportunities to put both kinds of improvements into effect.[71]

The environmentalists wished to modify the hospital to make it healthier. They would separate patients by disease, age, and sex, and create institutions specialising according to disease. They would also introduce ventilation devices for their capacity to disperse noxious odours believed to carry disease. To the environmentalist – who noticed that the diseased emit harmful effluvia – the hospital was a site of air loaded with disease matter. This is a territory at which traditional contagion and environmentalist theory most obviously merged.

The physician of the environment wished to remove the stench of sickness and of the congregation of unwashed bodies. Ventilators would drive this disease matter, which seemed to be both particulate and gaseous, away from the sick, the merely wretched, and the healthy. There is in this no clear anticipation of the present-day idea of air-borne contagion, specifically of disease-carrying droplets emitted by the infected and passed to the healthy.[72] Nevertheless once again we must suspect that a useful measure was introduced, if for reasons which at best are only partially correct. Ventilators – and more generally the shift from closed to open windows, from still to moving air – should be expected to have removed disease-carrying droplets from the air of hospitals, as well as from other public and private structures.

To establish the effects of ventilation and ventilators, improved and unimproved sites must be compared. Bisset Hawkins claimed in 1829 that hospital mortality in Britain had declined since the middle of the eighteenth century.[73] This he attributed to ventilation, greater cleanliness, and an improved standard of material comfort. McKeown suggests that maternal mortality may have declined in eighteenth-century England and Wales because hospitals were cleaned and ventilated.[74] More generally, the same source points out that air-borne diseases (that is, disease spread by droplets and dust) can be prevented by ventilation, and that this is especially significant wherever the uninfected are in close contact with the infected.[75]

Obviously, however, the expectations of the environmentalists for ventilation could not have been achieved. The disease of close quarters – malignant fever, probably typhus – is not transmitted by means that can plausibly be said to have been affected by ventilation. Quite the contrary. If the incidence of louse-borne typhus is associated with the infrequency with which people wash themselves and their apparel, and washing with ambient temperature, then ventilating hospitals, prisons, ships, and other sites would have lowered indoor temperatures and left individuals less inclined to wash or change clothes. Hence lice populations should be expected to have continued to thrive – deterred only, perhaps, by fumigations, such as by burning sulphur matches.

Where ventilation may have had a beneficial effect is rather with air-borne diseases, especially diptheria, influenza, measles, tuberculosis, and pneumonia (among major causes of death in the early modern era). But it should be remembered that this is the category of disease transmission – considering diseases transmitted by physical contact, water, food, insects, and fomites – before which public health measures have remained the least powerful up to the present. Infectious diseases transmitted by insects, food, and water have not for many decades been major causes of death. But the principal measures now used against air-borne diseases are immunological or chemotherapeutic. Ventilation is nevertheless a measure of distinct efficacy in certain circumstances, for moving air will more quickly dissipate droplet nuclei and carry air-borne pathogens out of crowded quarters. For the eighteenth century, however, its efficacy would seem to be limited to situations in which it was applied for the first time – not the house or tenement but the site of public gatherings or of people held, voluntarily or involuntarily, in close quarters, such as the ship or prison. Houses, still heated by wood or coal fires built in fireplaces, had their own ventilation systems in winter, as a result of the drawing action of fires.

Mortality at Sea

Ventilation and lavation may explain part or all of an observed decline in mortality on board ships. On slaving and other merchant vessels, and on naval vessels, mortality fell between about 1750 and 1825. Voyage-specific mortality on British slavers was, by 1810–40, less than half what it had been in the 1680s.[76] The chief causes of death on board French and British slavers were dysentery, yellow fever, unspecified fevers, smallpox, and measles.[77] That is to say, the diseases that cost slaves and slaver crews so heavily were air-, water-, and vector-borne. All may have been influenced by ventilation and lavation. Hales' ventilators were widely used on British merchant and slave ships, and in 1753 they were introduced into the French slave trade, reportedly with the effect that mortality fell.[78]

The same effect appears on merchant and naval vessels. Ventilation devices (especially Hales' windmill, which forced air into the ship's holds) were introduced on British navy vessels, including hospital and troop ships, beginning in the 1750s.[79] During the Seven Years' War Navy Board estimates indicate that 184 893 sailors and marines served on British ships.[80] Of that number, 1 512 died in combat or from accidents, and 133 708 men deserted, died from disease, or were discharged because of sickness. Stephen Gradish estimates the number of deserters at 40 000, meaning that upwards of 90 000 men died or were discharged for disease. Yet these figures amounted to fewer losses than suffered during the War of Austrian Succession in the 1740s. More specifically, the great typhus epidemic in the British navy in the 1740s was not repeated during the 1750s, suggesting that lice-borne infection had been curtailed (even though certainly not via ventilation). Furthermore, naval hospital cure rates improved dramatically during the 1750s and 1760s. At one naval hospital, located at Haslar, 9 862 of 14 418 admissions were cured during 1753–7. Gradish attributes this to isolation by disease and other improvements.[81] Of these numbers it should be remembered that the British navy recruited sailors chiefly from the merchant marine. These large numbers of sailors thus represent a labour force at sea in peace and war time.

Arthropod Vectors

Ventilation intruded upon air-borne disease but, Dobson's remarks about mosquitoes notwithstanding, probably had less effect on disease vectors than other measures. Certainly prison fever – epidemic typhus – will not have been reduced directly by ventilation, as Hales and Pringle believed. This variety is transmitted by the faeces of body lice, and other varieties are passed by similar vectors (mites and fleas) that would have been unaffected by the reduction of air-borne droplets which ventilation would have brought. Nevertheless, both the cleansing of the prison and the measures of antisepsis proposed by environmentalists may have driven lice and fleas away from man. Some historians have suggested this result.[82] Considering the problem of typhus from the perspective of 1829, Bisset Hawkins believed that it had diminished in incidence for exactly these reasons.[83] Although entomologists dismiss as useless most of the insecticides named in eighteenth-century literature, they acknowledge the effectiveness of burning sulphur and alkaloids, and of the mixture pyrethrum, which causes paralysis in flies and fleas and was first used in Europe in the early nineteenth century (and is still in use today).[84]

Among other insect vectors, those of chief importance are the fly and probably also the cockroach, which are called mechanical vectors because they pick up and distribute pathogens by accident and apparently play no biological role in pathogen development. Synanthropic flies (those which coexist with man) include the housefly and such common blowflies as the bluebottle and greenbottle. Feeding on refuse, faeces, decaying substances, and on human food, flies are known to carry stupendous numbers of pathogens, as also are cockroaches. The question is whether these insects play a large role in disease transmission.

In the modern developed world they clearly do not, for mechanical devices and insecticides diminish contacts between man and these arthropods, and refuse disposal and insect eradication programmes reduce their numbers. But the question is whether contacts between man and these vectors were much more common in the seventeenth century. Entomologists recognise that the factor of leading importance in the role of arthropods as vectors is numbers. Although each insect will, even in a clean environment, carry huge numbers of pathogens, contacts between these insects and man are haphazard. What is important is not the numbers of pathogens, which in any case may exceed a million per insect, but the numbers of the insects themselves.

In the pre-environmentalist era all the conditions of life seem to have been ideal for immense arthropod populations, especially in the late summer and early autumn. These insects breed in the greatest numbers where refuse, faeces, decaying matter, and the like are left undisposed, and therefore provide both sites to lay eggs and to feed. Flies are said to prefer horse manure over all other animal faeces, but to be particularly adept at finding sites for reproduction and feeding. The growth of livestock herds – which McNeill posits as a possible reason for the decline of malaria in Europe – and especially the replacement of oxen by horses as draft animals, may thus be expected to have added to early modern Europe's fly population. How strange it sounds to discuss the numbers of insects in the past. We cannot measure quantities even today. It is possible to trap some, thereby to gauge changes in relative density, and that is often done in areas where arthropods of any type are important disease vectors. Such measures show that outbreaks of diarrhoeal diseases are closely associated with heavy fly populations.[85] But of the pre-eighteenth-century population of flies, mosquitoes, lice, cockroaches, and other insects we know only that they were numerous. Entomologists, who emerged in the seventeenth century, poets, writers, and observers of nature mention their great numbers. And thus, on circumstantial rather than statistical grounds, and because diseases transmitted by these insects are believed to have been major causes of sickness and death then but are so no longer, these sources establish the likelihood that mechanical and biological arthropod vectors played a much larger role in European disease transmission in the seventeenth century than they have in the twentieth century. These vectors may be charged specifically with the transmission of some filth diseases, dysentery and typhoid (which are probably the leading causes of diarrhoeas among early modern infants and children), plus malaria, plague, and typhus.

Without understanding that insects might play a significant role in disease transmission, the environmentalist proposed measures likely to have sharply reduced breeding and feeding opportunities for some of these insects. Drainage, as has already been established, is the most effective means to reduce mosquito populations below the critical population density necessary to sustain the disease. The *Anopheles* strains thus survive in Britain and on the continent, but not in large enough numbers to pose a serious malarial threat to man. Lavation, fumigation and insecticides seem likely to have reduced Europe's lice population, thereby helping explain the declining importance of typhus as a cause of death by the nineteenth century. And, for unknown reasons, the flea's role in transmitting plague was disturbed in the latter decades of the seventeenth century, very probably in some manner unconnected to environmentalist remedies, which had not yet passed from the stage of theory to action.

Did the mechanical vectors experience changes similar to those of the mosquito and the louse? The diseases of greatest importance transmitted by the mechanical vectors are dysentery (amoebic and bacillary) and typhoid. These diseases may also be transmitted by contaminated food, amoebic dysentery also by water, and typhoid also by physical contact. No significant improvements in food handling or preservation, or in water purity, are known to have occurred before the second half of the nineteenth century. And, since environmentalist theory laid less stress on the dangers of contagion, there seems no reason to suspect any change in willingness to tolerate physical contact between people. The most likely area for change lies in the population of those insects commonly assigned responsibility for transmitting these diseases, especially the fly and the cockroach. In lavation and relocation, the environmentalists proposed measures that would diminish the number of breeding and feeding sites, and detach ramaining sites – the slaughterhouse, refuse pit, and cemetery all to be moved outside the town – from dense human populations.

If so much can be made of drainage, ventilation, and lavation as remedies likely to have reduced disease risks, can the same be said of reinterment? As many observers, most recently Michel Ragon, have noticed, man has long felt a desire to bury the dead and a sense that inadequate disposal of human remains might be dangerous, even fatal, to the living. Early modern Europeans on the continent lived amongst the dead, using cemeteries as sites for festivals and social gatherings, and visiting regularly the church housing the dead. The environmentalists asserted, citing specific cases, that proximity to the dead (and especially to the dead improperly buried) was epidemiologically dangerous. The living were at risk before the dead. They proposed to transfer existing remains and to relocate cemeteries outside the city.

Do the dead pose such a threat to the living? There is not, to all appearances, much research on this issue. The pathologist knows that cutting into the remains of someone who has died of certain diseases – tuberculosis for example – may be dangerous unless precautions are taken, and that anthrax and smallpox pathogens survive for some time in the dead. But more generally the pathogens that cause disease die with, or shortly after, their hosts, and pose little or no risk to the living. The microorganisms that develop in a dead body, one that has not been embalmed or eventually in one that has, are rarely pathogenic. Where the dead may pose a risk to the living is by serving as breeding and feeding ground for insects and rodents. Corpses buried in shallow graves are known to provide feeding opportunities for rodents, and certain synanthropic flies (especially bluebottles and greenbottles) are known to feed on decaying matter of many kinds, including animal and human corpses, beginning with the face. Remains improperly disposed of, those thrown casually into the large burial pits that served the urban poor and those disposed of hurriedly in shallow trenches during epidemics, may thus pose a significant indirect disease threat to the living by supporting abnormally high arthropod and rodent populations. In persuading governments across Europe to relocate cemeteries, and to dispose of the dead with greater care, the environmentalists mounted another unintentional attack on the arthropods.

In a general way the environmentalists' measures constituted an unwitting (but nonetheless potentially effective) attack on the breeding places and living sites of animate vectors which transmit disease. The refuse swept from streets and passages, the waste buried on land or deposited in the sea, the standing water, moat, and puddle drained, and other measures began to remove from man's habitat sites where houseflies, mosquitoes, rodents, and all manner of animate disease vectors thrive. Moreover, applied to hydraulic improvements, lavation also transformed the still waters of canals and cisterns into moving waters, thus making them less attractive to mosquitoes and other insects. This unwitting attack provides an explanation for the declining incidence of typhoid, which Rosen located in the latter part of the eighteenth century,[86] and for dysentery, malaria, and typhus. Indeed, plausibly, the appearance of cholera may be related not merely to the growth of large cities, which were not of course a new phenomenon in Europe, but to the success of the environmentalists' efforts. Lavation transferred the pathogen-laden refuse from the street to the river, and therefore shifted the site of contamination from the refuse pit to the water supply. The nineteenth-century cholera epidemics may therefore be an ironic measure of the success of the eighteenth-century campaign to avoid disease.

CONCLUSION

The medicine of the environment mounted a direct attack on sites and conjunctions of the habitat that seemed unhealthy, and on the emanations of these things and of the people made diseased by them. It did not recognise the existence of living disease vectors, specifically overlooking Lancisi's suggestion of animate carriers of malaria matter, and failing to suspect that the many insects, rodents, and other visible organisms that surrounded eighteenth-century man might play a large role in disease transmission. The attack on environmental pathogens we can recognise, however, as an unwitting attack on the living vectors of disease.

The argument developed here specifies Richard Shryock's claim, advanced in 1936, that the second half of the eighteenth century witnessed a renaissance in hygiene.[87] It was not the hygiene of the individual that was improved. It was instead the hygiene of site. The environmentalists' attack on those locations in the habitat from which disease seemed to spring constituted, we can see only in retrospect, an attack not against disease itself but against common disease carriers. It sought to remove stench, the most powerful sign of disease. In doing so, it had the effect of destroying sites in which thrive those insects and small animals which transmit disease. If we possessed an historiography of insects and rodents, we should expect it to treat the second half of the eighteenth century as the beginning of a great dark age.

7 Conclusion

> The *enquête* was unable not to find what it looked for.[1]
>
> Peter

In the medium run, in the second half of the nineteenth century, the idea of a pathogenic environment would give way to theories focusing on bacteriology and infective agents. In the longer run, the theory would be revived, although not from its mid-nineteenth-century form but from earlier, purer ideas about how environmental and meteorological forces influence health, and about the environment as host not so much to disease as to the living vectors that carry disease. In the short run, however, the medicine of the environment would continue to thrive during the first half of the nineteenth century, and for some learned medical scientists still two or three decades thereafter. The scope of this book ends around the turn into the nineteenth century, a time when – for most European physicians who reflected about epidemic disease – environmentalist thinking was orthodox thinking. In the eighteenth-century form of this idea the miasma theory is submerged in a host of ideas about the sources and causes of epidemics. In the nineteenth-century form, the notion of gaseous rather than particulate means of disease transmission, and of little other than miasmic means, would claim control. Ironically, a simpler theory would thus replace a more complex theory without undermining medical confidence in the efficacy of measures to treat the environment as a source of pathogens. The era of the cholera epidemics, roughly 1825–75, is a period of insistent cries for environmentalist remedies in the face of still greater problems posed by the sudden shift of urban populations toward rapid growth. Indeed most of the remedies credited with fashioning the late nineteenth-century part of Europe's long mortality decline remain, despite the interim formulation of the germ theory, the remedies of environmentalism.

Toward the end of the eighteenth century a number of physicians reasserted the relevance of other non-naturals than air, and thus of forces the importance of which environmentalism had discounted.[2] In the *Encyclopédie méthodique: médecine*, Jean-Noël Hallé, who had charge of instruction in hygiene in the new Parisian medical faculty organised in 1794, sought to redefine the non-naturals as 'matière de l'hygiène', and in the process to reabsorb neglected elements.[3] Others, especially M. F. B. Ramel, author of a study of the atmospheric constitution of the commune of Gemenos in the Bouches-du-Rhône, maintained specifically that modern medicine had carried too far the theory of emanations, and attributed too much significance to the idea that air harbours disease.[4] But in the main epidemiological theory continued to focus on air, and especially on its capacity to absorb and transmit miasmas.

To conclude, it may be useful to draw together several strains of this investigation in order to consider again how and why the theory of environmentalism so successfully resisted critical scrutiny in the eighteenth century. This is one of two issues for which a summing up is needed. The other – the hypothesis that environmental engineering contributed to the eighteenth- century regression of mortality – will follow.

THE HISTORY OF DISEASE THEORY

To organise this first part of the conclusion let me pose the discussion in terms of a debate that developed among physicians in Philadelphia in 1793. On 6 or 7 August of that year, a child in the family of Dr. Hodge died. In the weeks that followed more residents died with similar symptoms, and at the height of the epidemic, in September and early October, thousands more. In mid- or late October the epidemic waned, as cold and wet weather replaced warm and dry. According to the diagnosis finally accepted by the city's physicians, this was an epidemic of yellow fever, one of several in Philadelphia and other American seaports during the eighteenth century.[5]

Since 1900 yellow fever has been known as a mosquito-borne infection. It is endemic in tropical Africa and the Americas, but may occur in epidemic form in temperate regions during warm seasons.[6] The causal mechanism of the disease is now understood but, as James D. Goodyear has recently pointed out, its history is still an enigma.[7]

The question that most troubled physicians in Philadelphia dealt with the source of the epidemic. At the head of a group insisting that the yellow fever had not been imported but had arisen from factors present in the city stood Benjamin Rush, whose habit was to engage actively in public debate and to conduct the debate in a contentious manner. Rush argued that the general conditions necessary for the epidemic might be found in the environmental and epidemic constitution that preceded the outbreak. The specific and immediate cause he assigned to a cargo of damaged and putrescent coffee lying together with some other peccant substances on wharves above Arch Street.[8] In the literature taking Rush's side this explanation is often buttressed by citations of the case of a Mr Moore, an early victim who was known to have passed by those wharves and believed to have been taken ill by the stench, or by references to the cases of several sailors who were the first people exposed to the stench and among the first to become ill.

Rush's opponents constituted most of the members of the Philadelphia College of Physicians. Like some outspoken members of the populace, such as the Lutheran pastor Helmuth and the journalist Mathew Carey, these physicians argued that the disease had been imported from the West Indies and then transmitted by contagion.[9] Rush, too, at first wrote of contagion as a force in the spread of the disease,[10] but neither he nor his opponents clearly specified what they had in mind by the word 'contagion'. When his opponents argued that yellow fever had never been known to have arisen on its own in a North American city, Rush answered that in the West Indies, where the disease was know to be endemic, and in North America it arose from the same causes: the exhalations of putrid vegetable matter.[11] This argument depended on reports of the disease from the West Indies, where several environmentalist physicians (William Hillary, Richard Towne, Benjamin Moseley, John Hunter, and Robert Jackson, among others) had anticipated Rush's explanation of cause.[12] Rush later, in 1803, explained the points at issue more straightforwardly. Some fevers are contagious and are transmitted either by secretion (smallpox and measles) or excretion (jail fever), which transmit these diseases only at short distances.[13] Others are not contagious and spread only by means of 'exhalations from putrid matters'.[14] It is this circumstance that provides grounds for drainage and urban cleansing as devices of avoidance and prevention.

Despite some rancour in their disagreement on origin, there was a wide consensus among Philadelphia's physicians about public health measures to adopt to diminish the impact of the epidemic. Although Rush's opponents argued that the disease had appeared and been transmitted by contagion, they too turned to what were by 1793 standard remedies of enviromentalism such as street cleansing, hospital expansion, and ventilation.[15] Rush endorsed any measure that might diminish (or diminish contact with) vegetable putrefaction. He also railed against another standard public health measure of colonial American ports, the quarantine, which he maintained was ineffective and for that reason demoralising. Such an attitude, as Erwin Ackerknecht has shown, found favour both among businessmen (for whom quarantines meant economic losses) and among classical liberals (who objected to state interference and singled quarantines out as an example of the interference that should be ended). In 1793 this case was only beginning to gather momentum; by the 1820s and thereafter it would lead to changes in and the elimination of quarantine laws.[16]

In the realm of therapy the physicians of the city fell again into disagreement, and in the short run it seemed likely that Rush's case about the origin of the epidemic might be discredited for its association with the particularly aggressive therapy he adopted. William Cobbett, later editor of the aptly titled *Porcupine's Gazette* and fully Rush's equal in acerbity, compared mortality statistics during the epidemic to test whether Rush's method of treatment, which relied heavily on so-called heroic bleeding and purging, was effective. Cobbett concluded that Rush was a public menace and showed that the incidence of mortality had increased with the incidence of Rush's treatment.[17] By way of response, Rush argued vigorously in favour of his therapeutic programme, claiming that he and his pupils had cured fully ninety-nine of every hundred patients who came to them upon the first appearance of symptoms. In contrast at the hospital more than half the cases admitted ended in death.[18] A more persuasive defence against Cobbett's charges could have been mounted by observing that Cobbett had unreasonably overlooked the curve of the epidemic itself, which insured that mortality would continue to increase as long as the number of stricken grew. But Rush instead claimed a rate of cure that in restrospect can only seem incredible.

On their own, Rush's arguments about the epidemic and the proper therapeutic response to it might have fared poorly. But they harmonised with prevailing ideas about epidemic disease and its treatment – and, more to the point, they were buttressed by the case made in 1796 by the ship's surgeon James Bryce.[19] Bryce was uncertain about the method of the disease's transmission, but he reported the appearance of yellow fever on a vessel that had not since leaving England had any contact with other vessels or ports. The epidemic began as the ship passed the equator. Furthermore Bryce revealed that he cured nearly everyone stricken by the use of 'drastic purgatives'. These traditional remedies of humoural pathology were already viewed with scepticism by many physicians, but Bryce's epidemic history helped establish Rush's argument about the local origin of yellow fever.

In the meantime it was the 1793 debate that prompted Noah Webster to investigate the causes of epidemics in general. To that end he compiled *A Brief History of Epidemic and Pestilential Diseases*, which he expected both to determine the true causes of epidemics and to isolate effective remedies.[20] His study of a wide variety of authorities reporting on historical epidemics led Webster to conclude that epidemics are caused by pestilential constitutions of the atmosphere: 'All the great plagues that have afflicted mankind, have been accompanied with violent agitations of the [meteorological and geological] elements'.[21] He thus attributed the influenza of 1789 to a series of earthquakes in North America and to the eruption of Vesuvius on 29 October, which caused a darkness over Kentucky.[22] Although Rush was pleased with what he saw as Webster's presentation of his own case, the lexicographer's scheme drew criticism from other physicians. But the grounds for their objections to it had less to do with its environmentalist assertions and methodologies than with Webster's having stepped into a field with which he was not entirely familiar.

The case Rush made about the origin and transmission of yellow fever in 1793 and the case Webster made about the origin and transmission of most epidemic diseases (excepting, for example, smallpox)[23] in other times and places was, in its principal elements, the case of the medicine of the environment.

Epidemics are generated and transmitted by the confluence of certain physical forces. They may last longer than the confluence. They end when combatted by an antagonistic set of physical forces, like the cold and wet autumn in Philadelphia in 1793. There is much in this theory that is attractive, for the bacteria and infectious matter that are the immediate causes of disease are themselves influenced by the environment in which they exist. Eighteenth-century physicians noticed that some diseases, such as yellow fever, are seasonal. Of yellow fever they noticed also that it occurs chiefly among people living in low-lying areas, that contact with infected people at certain hours of dusk often leads to contraction of the disease, and that prior sufferers are immune.[24] Of course, they overlooked the intermediary roles of bacteria and infectious matter, and of the vectors that sometimes transmit diseases, including yellow fever. The things that they neglected prevented the development of a satisfactory understanding of the origin and transmission of disease. But the things they did notice, the procedure of surveillance that they recommended for disease and the environment, and the inferences they drew about how to disrupt the environment–disease association all constituted insights of considerable force, and perhaps also of considerable efficacy.

In Philadelphia, some physicians argued that the yellow fever had been brought to the port by a vessel from the West Indies. Superficially there is much in the contagion theory as advanced by the Philadelphia College of Physicians that appears to resemble or anticipate present-day ideas about the transmission of some diseases. But the contagion theory they advanced cannot be distinguished from the environmentalist view of disease transmission, for it had been subsumed by environmentalist theory. Rush did not represent the medicine of the environment and the College of Physicians did not represent a memory of earlier contagionist theory. They agreed on too many points. More to the issue at hand, Rush's 1803 explanation of disease transmission reveals that one environmentalist at least still believed that both particulate matter and vapour may play a role. The intriguing question raised by the debate of 1793, a question that we are now prepared to address, has to do not with why superior theories and therapies were not brought to bear in the eighteenth century, but with why an incomplete and inadequately tested theory of epidemic causation flourished. What was it about the medicine of the environment, this eighteenth-century variety of medical geography and biometeorology, that made it so persuasive for so long?

Thinking back over the contents of this book, it is evident that the answer has two parts. It arises, on the one hand, from the congruence of environmentalist thought with non-medical appreciations of man and man's world in the eighteenth century. It arises, on the other hand, from features peculiar to medical thought and practice.

The rich literature on eighteenth-century thought, especially works such as Glacken's study of man's views of nature, reveals an age in which nature was the particular object of curiosity. The thinkers of this age, whether professedly enlightened or not, demanded explanations of physical phenomena. Some expected to discover the intricacies of a world fashioned by a divine hand, the better to appreciate the majestic accomplishment of the deity; others concerned themselves more with the mechanics of a world that resembled a clock whose maker had created the instrument, wound it up, and then withdrawn. All expected to discover an orderly nature, a nature not only open to human understanding but also – to some degree at least – to human manipulation. At every turn man seemed to have run foul of this design, to have failed to multiply his numbers as rapidly as allowed by nature, to have failed to be as prosperous as might be, and to suffer many evidences of discord with nature, many unhappinesses. Epidemic desease was one of these signs of discord, for its existence revealed that man had not adjusted himself satisfactorily to his habitat. The eighteenth-century theory of nature held nature responsible for many of man's failures, but man responsible for taking those actions that would end the discord. Physicians shared these ideas, for the literature of environmentalism is full of assumptions that arise from this view of man's relationship with nature. To put the point another way, knowing what we know about non-medical thought in the eighteenth century, and called upon to guess the direction of medical thought, we should guess the existence of a medicine of the environment. In short, one reason this approach to the problem of health seemed so persuasive for so long is because it harmonised so well with the world view of other branches of curiosity.

What is to me more interesting is the second part of the answer to this question, the part that deals directly with medical issues. Here we penetrate beyond generally shared images, and investigate why a specific group accepted such images. In this realm, the answer lies in noticing that the theory of a pathogenic environment satisfied more of the available evidence about epidemic disease than did any alternative explanation. The environmentalist's scepticism about conventional contagion theory was well placed, for that theory did fail to explain how the same disease might appear simultaneously in widely separated locales. Moreover, beyond the quarantine, contagion theory relied on the efficacy of the physician's treatment of the individual patient. Practising physicians like Rush did not doubt the success of their own therapies, even though they often relied on therapies that to us seem unlikely to have had beneficial effects. But in the hands of other physicians, existing techniques – especially the heroic treatments used so freely by Rush in 1793 – did not seem to be so efficacious. Sydenham's search into case histories and the environmental constitution, and his recommendation that the physician's gaze fall on both the patient and the patient's habitat, constitute a response to the inefficacy of conventional theory and therapy. Later epidemiologists shifted more of their gaze on to the environment because there they hoped to find an efficacious large-group medicine. This direction of sight revealed a host of forces that might account for the puzzling appearance and disappearance of epidemics. And it had behind it the force of Hippocratic approval.

We must notice also that the medicine of the environment did not generate evidence that seemed to undermine its assumptions. This is so, in the first place, because the things in the environment being observed were numerous and often only vaguely differentiated. Perhaps the longest single list was provided by Thomas Short, but many environmentalists suggested additions to it, or fresh ideas about combinations within the existing list. And others, while not adding to the list of variables deemed relevant, did add to the volume of data available about one or more of these variables. In 1776 Vicq d'Azyr organized a comprehensive effort to gather data, hoping to build a comprehensive collection of the signs and signals of the environment. He wanted also to create an international community of physicians informed about these things, and about their meaning for the recognition and treatment of disease. The task of compilation was fulfilled. But the fulfilment of Boissier de Sauvages' suggestion to Jean Razoux (that for fifty years thirty physicians gather such data as Razoux had on Nîmes) and much more did not solve the problem of detecting or testing specific associations. Indeed it may have undermined it, for the data gathered in Vicq d'Azyr's *enquête* were so numerous that they may still defy analysis.[25] Not quite forty years after Boissier de Sauvages' remark (made in 1760) Jean Baptiste Demangeon foresaw a task still so formidable as to require the cooperation of laymen, and an arena so broad as to shove the issues merely of meteorology into the background.[26]

This endless expansion of the territory to be searched owes something to the mathematical technology of environmentalism and of the eighteenth-century investigation of man in general. According to the law of large numbers, discrepancies between reality and observations of reality would diminish as the number of observations grew. But this approach failed to indicate any point at which additional observations would cease to be useful, or sufficiently useful, to warrant their collection. The vast energy of the scientist of man was thus directed toward observation and away from hypothesis testing. Only the technique of sampling, a much later addition to the tools of statistics, would redirect this energy toward gathering the minimum amount of data necessary for a predetermined range of error.

Nor were the things observed adequately distinguished from one another. This problem of discrimination has two features. In one the physician, especially Short, seemingly named everything he could think of as a relevant variable. In the other, the physician failed to name distinct entities, or failed carefully to specify the nature of the thing being measured, such as happened in the case of air humidity. Or, on a variation on this theme, the physician possessed only imperfect instruments for measuring environmental forces. Different thermometers gave different readings in the same circumstances, a matter of considerable importance in a climate in which temperature variability is comparatively modest. Moreover, the things measured by other instruments, such as the eudiometer, were not always clear. Even if straightforward associations should exist between weather or climate and disease, the meteorologist-physician was thus ill prepared to detect them.

Each step toward adding new variables and away from precision and discrimination compounded the combinatorial problem, and further confounded the matter of specifying cause. This is so because each step added a new range of interactive influence between the new variable and some, or all, previously designated variables. Each step of this sort took the physician farther away from any possibility of testing environmentalist theory.

In the second place, the medicine of the environment did not produce evidence that tended to undermine its assumptions because the techniques available for detecting associations among these elements and factors, on the one side, and disease, on the other, were not adequate to the task. The eighteenth-century medical statistician anticipated a mathematics of correlation, which would not appear until the end of the nineteenth century. What is more, the associations that the environmentalists seemed to detect by viewing the data on disease and the habitat often appeared to be variable rather than fixed. The wet and cold autumn did not always end a prevailing epidemic, as it appeared to do in Philadelphia in 1793. Medicine had absorbed the objective of eighteenth-century science and given itself over to the collection of data about the world. David Rittenhouse and several other Philadelphians thus kept meteorological journals during the 1793 epidemic. Rittenhouse's readings of barometric pressure, temperature, wind direction, and general weather for August until 9 November were published by Carey on 23 November.[27] Like so many other meteorological–disease records, they revealed a unique pattern. A better grasp of combinatorial mathematics would have suggested that nothing else should be expected when so many phenomena were being observed.

But the medical statistician lacked this insight. The problem at hand thus became more complex for – recognising the variability of the mechanism of causation or influence – the environmentalist elected to search further into the habitat for the elements explaining this variability. Environmental theory had adjusted to its failure to detect fixed associations by positing that different atmospheric and environmental constitutions could produce the same epidemic constitution. It is here that the force of the argument from analogy becomes evident. Reasoning from analogous cases involved an assumption about the power of analogy to explain. One may recognise the force of analogy to teach – that is, to explain things known by other means. But the existence of an analogous relationship between two things no longer seems a persuasive reason to draw conclusions about things not known from things known, or believed to be known.

At the heart of matters, the technique of environmentalism consisted not of observation, aggregation, and induction, but of observation, aggregation, and inference from analogy. And because reasoning from analogy figured so prominently in its methodology, environmentalism's frame of reference continued to be dominated by old patterns of thought, to which analogies were drawn. When Montesquieu studied the papillae of the sheep, he used that experiment to confirm an inference about sensibility and climate. In reality, however, he inferred that the experiment confirmed his view of climate and sensibility not because the experiment demonstrated what he said it did, but because he expected it to, and failed to see that it did not. The eighteenth-century physician lacked a means to determine whether a particular analogy was sound – or, to put it another way, lacked the means to test hypotheses.[28] Or, to be more precise, this physician lacked a sense of the need to test analogies and hypotheses. However, even if environmentalists had clearly seen the desirability of testing hypotheses, they lacked the mathematical technology necessary to do so in the complex combinatorial setting of mature environmental theory.

Third, the environmentalist search failed to produce the evidence that would undermine it because, as we now know, the things that were not detected – specifically germs and their vectors – did not lurk in the environment in any way that they might have been detected by the things the environmentalists did. Rush noticed in 1793 that 'moschetoes' were 'uncommonly numerous'.[29] But environmentalist theory regarded these things as irrelevant except insofar as insects added animal matter to the putrefying substances in the environment.

In the short run, Rush's explanation of the yellow fever epidemic of 1793 and of the appropriate regimen of treatment seemed in danger of rejection. But other research appeared to verify it. In 1855 René La Roche, briefly the authoritative theorist on yellow fever, followed Rush's explanation.[30] As is now known, this disease is transmitted from person to person by the bite of *Aëdes aegypti*, which has already bitten a victim and lived long enough for the virus to make its way from the mosquito's stomach to its salivary glands. It is not caused by contagion, and thus Rush and others were accurate in observing that people attending the sick rarely if ever became sick themselves.[31] In short, both Rush and the College of Physicians seem now to have been wrong. Yellow fever reveals the complexity of the problem of creating a single theory of disease origins.

While the medicine of the environment failed to explain epidemic disease, it did succeed in providing an explanation consistent with more of the known evidence than could be accounted for by other theories. Humoural pathology explained both individual and large-group manifestations of disease according to the balance (or imbalance) of certain forces within the patient. It also incorporated a certain view of some environmental factors as external influences – the non-naturals – which might provoke or provide the occasion for disease. Oriented toward the individual manifestation of disease, humoural pathology stressed idiosyncracy and uniqueness rather than commonality. And it propagated an array of therapies and regimens of doubtful value. In contrast, environmentalism diverted the physician's attention toward a combination of therapy, avoidance, and prevention. It proposed to treat the environment as well as the patient.

Similarly the environmental hypothesis accommodated more of the known facts of large-group disease than did sixteenth-century contagion theory. C. E. A. Winslow once argued that Sydenham's 'almost complete neglect of contagion as a practical factor in the spread of epidemic disease and. . .major stress upon the metaphysical factor of epidemic constitution held back epidemiological progress for two hundred years'.[32] But in fact the elements of a germ theory were not, as Winslow supposed,[33] at hand. It is an error to assume that contagionists in Sydenham's day meant by that term much the same thing as late nineteenth-century contagionists. Indeed in Sydenham's day contagion theory was vague. Environmentalism absorbed parts of it, adding them to what it deemed the relevant factors and forces of the habitat. In the process it offered a coherent theory of epidemic propagation that purported to explain the simultaneous appearance of the same epidemic in different locales, the development of yellow fever on Bryce's ship long at sea, and other instances of disease unaccountable in the conventional contagion theory. And, in the eighteenth century, this theory brought together the ideas of miasmic and particulate transmission of disease. Only in the nineteenth century would the focus fall chieflly on one of these.

THE SOCIAL HISTORY OF DISEASE

Between 1670 and 1750, the crude death rate in Europe began to decline, falling from a range of 25 to 40 per 1 000 per annum to less than 10 per 1 000 in the late twentieth century. This decline – one of the powerful factors behind modern population growth and one of the most noteworthy features of modern history – was distributed, sometimes unevenly, over the entire period from 1750 or earlier to the present. How is it to be explained? A convincing single explanation has never been offered. Most attempts to provide explanations speak to circumstances highly specific in time and limited in geographical range. The most puzzling part of the mortality decline is that situated before the nineteenth century. Hypotheses framed to account for mortality decline before 1800 – nutritional improvements, specific medical advances such as smallpox inoculation, and others–fail because they are limited in time or place, or because they conflict with economic evidence, especially price data. Some authorities have suggested that public health reconstrued – taken to include public and private actions on a broad front – may provide part or all of a successful explanation of pre-1800 mortality decline.

But what exactly constituted public health action in the eighteenth century? The answer lies chiefly, although not exclusively, in environmentalism. In the eighteenth-century conception, much influenced by Hippocratic thinking, public health reforms focused on efforts to cleanse the environment, to reduce its pathogenic properties and its capacity to promote epidemics. The medicine of the environment subjected man's habitat and its diseases to the physician's surveillance and sought, sometimes in alliance with economic motives and sometimes for public health reasons alone, to show mankind how to avoid disease. Its principal measures were drainage, lavation, ventilation, and reinterment, but these were joined by other remedies, including fumigation, refuse burial, relocation of refuse-producing industries and waste sites, and such hydraulic improvements as cleaner wells and equipment designed to keep water in motion.

To show that these measures worked, eighteenth-century environmentalists compared improved and unimproved sites, consistently reporting greater healthiness after improvement. A more rigorous test of one measure, drainage, has been provided in Dobson's comparison of mortality in sites before and after drainage. Although the tests agree, they are not numerous. Nor is it reasonable to suppose that a rigorous battery of tests can now be performed, given the incomplete nature of surviving information about eighteenth-century population, mortality and improvements. Like the other explanations offered for Europe's mortality decline, the evidence about environmentalist action is circumstantial. But it is richer and more compelling than the evidence for any other explanation.

This is so especially because environmentalism constituted a general attack against epidemic disease, and epidemics are observed to have occurred less frequently and to have been less severe as the mortality decline progressed. Epidemics, so common in the seventeenth century, and so important a feature of mortality in Europe, became less frequent during the eighteenth and nineteenth century. Those that did occur, including the nineteenth-century cholera and the 1918 influenza epidemics, carried off smaller average portions of the population. The phenomenon of death was changing. No longer were its causes primarily infectious diseases. No longer were children and young adults dying in such high proportions. And no longer was death able to conscript like a levy en masse.

The environmentalists intended that their measures of engineering and cleansing would drive from man's habitat many of the stenches and meteorological complexes that this medical theory associated with the onset of epidemics. In retrospect, we can see that stench is not a reliable sign of pathogens, that the environmentalists failed still to understand the origin of diseases and the modes of their transmission. Environmentalism had therefore an unwitting effect. It began to cleanse man's habitat of breeding and feeding sites for those insects and small animals that are the vectors of many diseases important in the European mortality structure before these improvements were adopted. Thinking merely about the surroundings of man before environmentalist treatment, we can recognise in them all the signs of a habitat ideally suited, within the temperature ranges of Europe, to sponsor dense insect and rodent populations. For both biological and mechanical vectors, the issue of chief importance is population density in proximity to man. Without suspecting that insects or small animals play a significant role in disease transmission, the environmentalists proposed measures that, in cleansing the habitat of breeding and feeding sites, must have substantially reduced the pest population.

To be sure, this was a large task, one not quickly completed. The eighteenth-century campaign did not eliminate the pests of mankind. Environmentalist improvements did not withstand natural disasters, as the sudden but short-lived reappearance of epidemic malaria in Denmark after the flood of 1825 demonstrates.[34] Literature on urban sanitation in the nineteenth century leaves this matter in no doubt. But the same literature shows that progress had been made, that portions of Paris' sewers had been walled in, that the European city had assumed responsibility for collecting and disposing of waste (even if it did not always live up to that responsibility), that swamp drainage and hydraulic engineering more generally were making headway, and that especially in the town and the village and in middle and upper class urban neighborhoods, the habitat of man had been cleansed.[35] What must be kept in mind is the radical discontinuity of nineteenth-century urban growth, following a long period of slow growth, or none at all, in urban populations. It was in the nineteenth century, after 1815, that the Thames became contaminated; in the eighteenth century it is believed to have been more or less as clean as it is in the late twentieth century. Urbanisation and industrialisation compounded the problems associated with environmental cleanliness. If the eighteenth-century mortality decline slowed between about 1820 and 1870, as it did, then this may be explained by the growth of cities and industries. What is surprising is that the mortality rate did not, in such circumstances, rise. An underlying trend decline, established in the eighteenth century, was sustained in the face of nineteenth-century urban growth. The nineteenth-century environment was not clean, and some filth diseases, such as cholera transmitted by contaminated water, continued to play a large role in European mortality. But the death rate from infectious diseases in general was shrinking before the nineteenth century began, and it was shrinking specifically in the realm of diseases transmitted by living vectors.

Environmentalist remedies aimed to make the habitat healthier.

If they succeeded in reducing mortality rates, then they may be expected also to have reduced morbidity. Environmentalist thinking did not distinguish between often fatal and seldom fatal diseases, although diseases with high case fatality rates naturally received more medical attention. Given the nature of environmentalist remedies, the most plausible view is that these measures diminished the incidence of a variety of diseases with low and high case fatality rates, that they reduced the rate at which single and overlapping diseases afflicted mankind, thereby contributing both to greater vigour in the population and to a lower incidence of risk to disease. If the environmentalist explanation is persuasive, morbidity trends should have declined more or less in tandem with mortality rates. Such a proposition cannot be tested until we obtain evidence about morbidity rates.

The eventual explanation for Europe's mortality decline will summon up a variety of forces to account for different phases of this long movement. Even for specific parts, it may be necessary to point to several factors rather than one. The eighteenth-century portion of this decline may thus be accounted for by some factors of clearly limited applicability, such as nutritional improvements, and by others of more general range, such as the environmentalist remedies, which were widespread in Europe and the European world. What is most satisfying about the environmentalist explanation is that it offers a way to reintroduce medicine, and human action, into the formula. For an age in which expectations about progress and about the efficacy of human action were as high as they were in the eighteenth century, it is pleasing to find a territory in which intervention seems to have worked. And how characteristics of the eighteenth century to find that territory in a realm in which useful measures were taken for the wrong reasons.

Notes and References

Footnotes will provide the author's last name, the date of publication, and (where appropriate) a page reference. Most seventeenth- and eighteenth-century sources are cited from original or early editions, but where recent (often annotated) editions have been issued I have used those and cited them under the name of the editor. The original author is then designated in parentheses. Initial publication dates are also given in parentheses for pre-1800 works for which subsequent editions were consulted.

INTRODUCTION

1. Mattock and Lyons, eds (Hippocrates), 1969, p. 2.
2. Winslow, 1952, p. 23.
3. Greenwood, 1953, p. 503.
4. It is, however, easy to exaggerate the contrast between the Hippocratic and Galenic traditions. As will become evident in Chapter 1, the environmentalists concerned themselves with one of the Galenic non-naturals, air. Sargent, 1982, p. xxvii, detected this also. In this instance, as in the case of contagion theory (which will be discussed below) an alternative theory was subsumed and integrated rather than abandoned.
5. Armengaud, 1973, p. 22; Reinhard *et al.*, 1968, p. 680.
6. See especially Reinhard *et al.*, 1968, *passim*; Dupâquier, 1979, pp. 9, 11, 34, 81; Blayo, 1975, pp. 128ff.; Wrigley and Schofield, 1981, *passim*; Flinn, 1981; Kunitz, 1983, pp. 349–64; McKeown, 1976, p. 43 and *passim*. On the relative weight of increased fertility v. decreased mortality in overall English population growth, see McKeown, 1978, pp. 536–7; Wrigley and Schofield, 1981, especially pp. 244–5.
7. Carmichael, 1983, respectively pp. 256, 264.
8. See especially Eyler, 1979, pp. 97–122 and *passim*; Coleman, 1982; Eyler, 1973, pp. 79–100; Lilienfeld, ed., 1980, summarising the essays by Eyler and Lilienfeld and Lilienfeld; Hannaway's discussion of the Lilienfeld and Lilienfeld essay in ibid., pp.

39–42; La Berge, 1977, 279–301; Hardy, 1984, 250–82; and, in the literature of the day itself, Hirsch, 1883–6.
9. Haviland, 1855; Hirsch, 1883, I, p. v; Dewhurst, 1963, p. 295.
10. Henschen, 1966, p. xiii.
11. Foucault, 1973, p. 51.
12. Jordanova, 1979, p. 119. However, Jordanova uses this phrase in a more restricted sense, to refer to how geological, geographical, and meteorological forces have at times been cited to explain the origins of disease.
13. Bynum, 1980, p. 225 and n. 63.
14. Shryock, 1936; Ackerknecht, 1948; Ackerknecht, 1967; Foucault, 1973; and Vess, 1975.

1 THE REVIVAL AND REFINEMENT OF HIPPOCRATIC IDEAS

1. Huxham, 1759–67, II, p. ii; Arbuthnot, 1733, pp. vi–vii.
2. E.g., Sloane, 1707–25, I, p. xvii. The introduction of 154 folio pages contains a lengthy treatment of the environment and diseases of Jamaica.
3. Mattock and Lyons, eds (Hippocrates), 1969, pp. 5–10, 92–116; Chadwick and Mann, eds (Hippocrates), 1950, 29–80; Sargent, 1982, 49–61.
4. Mattock and Lyons, eds (Hippocrates), pp. 42, 44.
5. Ibid., pp. 48–68, the quote from p. 60.
6. Arbuthnot, 1733, p. 154. See also ibid., p. 166, for Arbuthnot's variation on this.
7. Smith, 1979, pp. 19–20. Also Lonie, 1981, pp. 113–50.
8. Mattock and Lyons, eds (Hippocrates), 1969, p. 2,n.1.
9. Hull, ed. (Petty), 1963–4 reprint, I, p. 244, written between 1671 and 1676. 'Not yet very usual. . .' because Petty had been preceded by Graunt. Wilcox, ed. (Graunt), 1939.
10. Petty, 1755 (first published 1699), p. 49.
11. See especially Hacking, 1975; Maistov, 1974.
12. Riley, 1985, p. 4 and n.l.
13. Ibid., pp. 22–3.
14. On these inventions see Khrgian, 1970, pp. 21–76; Middleton, 1964; Middleton, 1969; Hellman, 1914–22, I, pp. 139–47; Frisinger, 1977, especially pp. 47–122. 'Climate' deals with the general pattern of weather (or short-term) phenomena, and is used in that meaning here rather than in the seventeenth-century sense of an area of latitude.
15. See Khrgian, 1970, pp. 34–8.
16. Pascal, regarded as the founder of hydrostatics, also organised

the first series of instrumental observations. Edmund Halley, who contributed very significantly to the assemblage of demographic data, was also an active meteorologist, among other interests. Christiaan Huygens also observed weather phenomena, and Robert Hooke was a weather historian. The non-instrumental observation of weather in a time series dates to at least as early as the late sixteenth century.

17. Boyle, 1666, pp. 186–9; and idem, 1692, which includes some of Locke's meteorological records. See also Halley's report on an investigation seeking associations between barometric readings and weather in Halley, 1686, pp. 104–16.
18. Glacken, 1967, p. 494 for the quote, pp. 425–7, and *passim*. Also Thomas, 1983, pp. 242–3 and *passim*.
19. Riley, 1985, pp. 17ff.
20. Glacken, 1967, p. 495.
21. Porter, 1980, p. 298.
22. Bourde, 1967, II, p. 1 077.
23. Dewhurst, 1966, pp. 60–7; and idem, 1963, pp. 6, 18–19, 37ff. and *passim*. See also Keele, 1974, pp. 240–8. Edmund Halley should be added to this group.
24. See the discussion of Boyle's ideas which follows.
25. Dewhurst, 1966, pp. 64–5; and – for extended discussion of Sydenham's concept of constitution and of the causes of fever epidemics – Greenwood, 1918–19, pp. 57–76; Bates, 1975, pp. 63–140. Also Sargent, 1982, pp. 129–59; Miller, 1962, pp. 129–40; King, 1970, pp. 113–33, especially pp. 121–3.
26. Here Boyle especially was giving direction to an otherwise old but inchoate interest in man and the climate. On literature in this area since the Renaissance, see Glacken, 1967, pp. 431–60.
27. E.g., Boyle, 1692; and Locke's own observations, in Locke, 1705.
28. Latham, ed. (Sydenham), 1848–50, I, pp. 41–238.
29. Ibid., I, pp. 32–3.
30. Bates, 1975, p. 158. See also the discussion of Greenwoods' views by E. W. Goodall in Greenwood, 1918–19, p. 70.
31. I understand Sydenham to have these three varieties of constitution in mind: atmospheric, where the influence of weather and climate are felt; environmental, where Sydenham adds Boyle's idea of unknown forces, hypothetically emanations from certain sources; and epidemic, which is the result but also still a complex rather than a simple construct. Bates and Greenwood, the authoritative interpreters of Sydenham, do not qualify Sydenham's various uses of the term 'constitution', but they do adopt schemes with which my distinctions are sympathetic. Both also stress 'the essential ambiguity of much [that] Sydenham advanced', to use a phrase from Greenwood, 1918–19, p. 64.

32. Latham, ed. (Sydenham), 1848–50, I, pp. 33, 100. Also Boulton, 1724, for a further development of the doctrine of emanations.
33. Lépecq de La Clôture, 1778, 2 vols in 1 076 pages. As appears in textual and footnote references to Sydenham, Sydenham's ideas and methods were much in the minds of French physicians before and after the 1784 translation of the relevant works by A. F. Jault.
34. Latham, ed. (Sydenham), 1848–50, I, pp. 239, 240. Also Bates, 1975, pp. 106ff. 134.
35. E.g., Latham, ed. (Sydenham), 1848–50, I. pp. 242, 243ff.
36. Dewhurst, 1963, p. 301. Also Poynter, 1973, pp. 223–34.
37. Sauvages [de la Croix], 1754 (first published 1753), pp. 19, 40.
38. Le Brun, 1778 (first published 1776), pp. 7–8.
39. Retz, 1784a (first published 1779), pp. 150–5, gives a good treatment of the eighteenth-century theory of the miasma.
40. Ibid., p. 87. Here Retz echoed Wintringham on contagious diseases. Wintringham, 1752, I, p. 180.
41. A long but sporadic interest is suggested by the irregular appearance of editions of relevant Hippocratic works, and also by the publications of a number of physicians relating epidemic disease to weather and environment. Among writers in that vein were Giovanni Filippo Ingrassia (1510–80), Hippolytus Guarinonius (1571–1654), and Guillaume de Baillou (1538–1616). See also Miller, 1962, p. 133 n. 15;Voigt, 1939, pp. 6–7; Smith, 1979, pp. 18–20.
42. See Koller, 1937, pp. 65–102.
43. Green and Grose, eds (Hume), 1964, respectively, I, pp. 246, 244.
44. I am offering a simplified explanation of prior ideas about disease causation. For a detailed survey of these intricate and abstract notions, see King, 1970, pp. 30–7 and *passim*. Also Greenwood, 1953, pp. 501–7, places late seventeenth-century views in a longer-term context.
45. Glacken, 1967, p. 12.
46. The Galenic non-naturals were: air, food and drink, movement and rest, excreta and retenta, sleep and wakefulness, and emotions. King, 1970, p. 34; Rather, 1968, pp. 337–47.
47. Arbuthnot, 1733, p. 156.
48. Latham, ed. (Sydenham), 1848–50, I, p. 100.
49. Rosen, 1958, p. 106.
50. Ibid.
51. E.g., Rush, 1793–1809, IV, pp. 54–5, discussing how he developed some symptoms of yellow fever while visiting a patient.
52. Wintringham, 1752, I, p. 1.
53. Ibid., I, p. 179.
54. Ibid., I, p. 180. But not all emanations suspended in the air seemed harmful. E.g., Banau, 1786, p. 8.

55. See Bisset, 1762, preface, for an unambiguous statement on this.
56. Arbuthnot, 1733, p. 187.
57. Ibid., pp. 180–2, citing Boyle (p. 181, n.).
58. Ibid., p. 191. Also Pointer, 1738 (first published 1723), p. 134: 'For Contagion is produc'd by an Efficient Cause; which. . .is either a Venomous Putrefaction or Pestilential Infection of the Air, which acts Internally and Externally upon a Human Body'; [Astruc], 1721, pp. 98–105, singling out heat and humidity as factors aiding the propagation of the plague.
59. Arbuthnot, 1733, p. 181.
60. It will be noticed that neither the contagion nor the environmental theory coped adequately with the problem of why some people do not contract the disease during an epidemic. That problem was construed to belong to the realm of individual rather than large-group phenomena, in which case humoural pathology could be pressed into service. E.g., Devèze, 1794, pp. 20, 22.
61. Notice the reaffirmation of this doctrine, traced especially to Boyle, in the article 'Emanations' in the *Encyclopédie*. It was written by d'Alembert.
62. In 1711 Lancisi had written a history of the 'rheumatic epidemic' in Rome in 1709 which seems to have been his first excursion into environmentalism. He had earlier (in *De Subitaneis Mortibus*) acknowledged the influence of weather on disease while emphasising humoral concepts. White and Boursy, eds and trans. (Lancisi), 1971, pp. 89–90; Ackerknecht, 1945, p. 43.
63. On the place of this map in the history of medical cartography, see Jarcho, 1970, p. 132.
64. Wintringham, 1718, announced his adherence to environmentalism.
65. Huxham, 1759–67 (first published beginning in 1739), which carries his observations from 1728–48. The dedication to this edition also mentions observations of 1724–7. A third volume, carrying observations onward from 1748, appeared posthumously in 1770.
66. Jurin, 1723, pp. 422–7.
67. Ker, 1746, I, pp. 77–96.
68. In addition to translating Huygens' *De Ratiociniis in ludo aleae* into English (with additions) as *Of the Laws of Chance*, Arbuthnot published (1710–12) 'An Argument for Divine Providence, Taken from the Constant Regularity Observ'd in the Births of Both Sexes', which is an argument for design based on vital statistics rather than on the more typical astronomical observations.
69. Aitken, 1892, pp. 409–35, reprints this essay, which appeared first in 1701.
70. Two later editions were also published (in London, 1751 and

1756), and there were also translations into French (Paris, 1742), and Latin (Naples, 1753). For a contrary view of Arbuthnot's genius see LeFanu, 1972, pp. 320–21; and for a balanced appraisal, Beattie, 1935.

71. Hales, 1731 (2nd edn, first published 1731), I, p. 358.
72. Arbuthnot, 1733, p. ix.
73. This is probably the 1705 dissertation by J. B. Hoffstadt for which Friedrich Hoffman served as praeses.
74. Among the continental environmentalists who elaborated on their debt to Arbuthnot, and usually to the French translation of his *Essay*, were Sarcone, 1770–2 (first published 1765), I, p. 20; Behrends, 1771, e.g., p. 83; Retz, 1784a (first published 1779), pp. 173ff. Glacken, 1967, p. 563; Dedieu, 1970 reprint, pp. 204–25, discuss Montesquieu's debt to Arbuthnot (really, Glacken writes, to Hippocrates).
75. Arbuthnot, 1733, respectively Chapters 2 and 3, pp. 22–68.
76. Ibid., respectively pp. 64, 67.
77. Ibid., p. 69.
78. Ibid., p. 141.
79. Ibid., p. 223.
80. Ibid., pp. 67, 193–200.
81. Ibid., pp. 194–200.
82. Greenwood, 1948, p. 53. Also G. Jones, 1956, pp. 149–58.
83. 1749.
84. Short, 1750, p. xii, for the quote, and pp. xii–iv for the rest. Most environmentalists excluded meteors and comets, but Short was not alone in adhering to the traditional view of these phenomena as fiery emanations from the earth. E.g., Pointer, 1738 (first published 1723), p. 131.
85. Short, 1750, p. xiv.
86. Ibid., p. 109.
87. Ibid., pp. 13–19.
88. Ibid., p. 163.
89. Short, 1767, pp. 21–2, 161–213.
90. Ibid., p. 20.
91. Ibid., *passim*; Short, 1750, *passim*.

2 MEDICAL GEOGRAPHY AND MEDICAL CLIMATOLOGY

1. Menuret de Chambaud, 1797, p. 100; Audin-Rouvière, 1793–4, p. 11, respectively.
2. E.g., Voigt, 1939, pp. 6, 10.

3. W. Wright, ed. (Ramazzini), 1964 reprint, pp. v, vi.
4. Ibid., p. xviii.
5. Ibid., pp. xviii–xxii, 527. The series stopped in 1694 because for a few years there were no epidemics at Modena, and Ramazzini became interested in barometric experiments and the study of occupational disease.
6. Ibid., pp. xxxi–ii. On the winter see also Haeser, 1839–41, II, pp. 250–2; Duyn, 1744.
7. King, 1970, pp. 182–203; King, ed. (Hoffmann), 1971a, pp. xiii–ix, discuss Hoffmann's corpuscular theory.
8. Hoffman, 1701. Dedicated to Leibniz.
9. Hoffman, 1705. Also Riley, 1985, p. 158n69. This *Dissertation* was translated into English and published with Ramazzini's *On the Diseases of Artificers* in 1746 as *A Dissertation on Endemial Diseases. Only Hoffman was identified as the author.*
10. Fischer, 1965 reprint, I, p. 296.
11. E.g., Schroeck, 1696, pp. 137–52.
12. King, ed. (Hoffmann), 1971a, p. 1.
13. Ibid., pp. 43–7; King, 1970, pp. 184–93.
14. King, ed. (Hoffmann), 1971a, pp. 45, 104. Also Kaiser, 1969, p. 1 062, whose lead quotation illustrates this preoccupation; and Lonie, 1981, pp. 113–50, who develops in detail Hoffmann's mechanism, which is an aspect of his understanding of disorder in the individual rather than of epidemic disease.
15. King, 1970, pp. 181–3.
16. As Manley, 1952, p. 300, has noticed, a number of Boerhaave's students and students of his students studied weather–disease associations. Also Lindeboom, 1968, pp. 355–74, on Boerhaave's international impact. Lépecq de La Clôture, 1776, *passim*, in an important French statement on the merits of environmental pathology, cites Boerhaave as belonging to this tradition.
17. E.g., Millar, 1779, p. 13.
18. E.g., Behrends, 1771, p. 83; and the *arrêt* of 1776 providing for a general medico–topographical inquiry in France. Meyer, 1972, p. 13.
19. Huxham, 1759–67, II, pp. ii–iii, cites Ramazzini and Hoffmann as inspirers.
20. Voigt, 1939. See also Philipsborn, 1949, pp. 776–9; Brügelmann, 1975, 131–49; Oberholzer, 1966. While extensive, Voigt's is not a comprehensive list. See also the collection of early titles in Sydenham, 1769, II, *passim*.
21. King, ed. (Hoffmann), 1971a, p. 45.
22. Voigt, 1939, pp. 23–4; Burggrave, 1751, pp. 60ff.
23. Under the title *Die göttliche Ordnung in den Veränderungen des menschlichen Geschlechts*.

24. Behrends, 1771, pp. 3–17 of the tables, and 16–17.
25. Ibid., p. 53.
26. Ibid., pp. 73ff.
27. Behrends was particularly impressed by J. G. Zimmermann's study of the physiological and psychological effects of wind.
28. Ibid., pp. 102–22.
29. Ibid., pp. 155ff.
30. Voigt, 1939, pp. 22–82; Haeser, 1882, III, pp. 448–591.
31. Rosen, 1946, pp. 527–38, translates the introduction to vol. III.
32. On which see Lesky, ed. (Frank), 1976; Rosen, 1953a, pp. 21–42; idem, 1953b, pp. 186–93.
33. Lesky, ed. (Frank), 1976, pp. 177–8.
34. 'I was induced to undertake the troublesome and difficult task of collecting and publishing a concise and faithful account of the Climates and Diseases of the United States of America, by a desire of removing the trouble and inconvenience which result from accommodating the rules of practice and forms of prescription made in other countries to the diseases which occur in this'. Currie, 1972 (first published 1792), p. 1. See also M. Jones, 1967, pp. 254–66, for a collection of comments by European travellers in North America about climatic and geographical influences on disease.
35. Lining, 1753, p. 284.
36. Chalmers, 1776, I, p. iii.
37. Currie, 1972 (first published 1792), p. 2 and *passim*.
38. Lind, 1777 (first published 1768); idem, 1779 (first published 1757). Also J. Clark, 1792 (first published 1773); R. Thomas, 1790; Rodschied, 1796; Dazille, 1785.
39. Lind, 1777 (first published 1768), p. 167.
40. Most notably, G. van Doeveren, who had written on Groningen. De Vooys, 1951, pp. 1–8, discusses Dutch medical geography toward the end of the eighteenth century, stressing the importance of foreign influences.
41. Van den Bosch, 1778, p. 11, these among a vast number of authorities cited throughout the text.
42. Ibid., pp. 130–264. Van den Bosch's consultants included L. P. van de Spiegel, then a local office holder in the province of Zeeland but to be *raadpensionaris* of the province of Holland.
43. Also Retz, 1784a (first published 1779), on the Low Countries in general.
44. Boix y Moliner, 1716.
45. Thiéry, 1791.
46. E.g., Blom, 1783.
47. E.g., Erndtel, 1730.
48. Russell, 1756.

49. E.g., Van den Bosch, 1778.
50. Moheau, 1778, pt. 1, pp. 22, 139–43, pt. 2, pp. 25ff. and *passim.* On Moheau's work, which is sometimes attributed to Montyon, see Coleman, 1977, pp. 101–8.
51. It should be noticed also that environmentalism penetrated veterinary medicine in France. For example, Jean Jacques Paulet considered the influence of harmful properties of the atmosphere in epizootics but rejected that as less likely than the conventional contagion hypothesis of direct transmission from animal to animal. Paulet, 1775, II, pp. 435ff. On the other hand, Paulet ascribed at least fifteen of every twenty serious epizootics to standing waters. Ibid., II, p. 440.
52. [Mairan], 1743, pp. 20–9; Malouin, 1746, pp. 220–54; Deparcieux, 1746, pp. 69–70; Vetter, 1975, pp. 347–67. See also the extended review of George Cleghorn's *Observations on the Epidemical Diseases in Minorca* in the *Journal des sçavans*, July 1756, pp. 281–302. The reviewer recommends Cleghorn's theory and method for French emulation.
53. E.g., Lépecq de La Clôture, 1776, p. xv.
54. 1767.
55. Razoux cites Hoffmann as a precursor (Razoux, 1767, pp. 6–7), but does not mention any others, and (p. 5) expresses the notion that he has been the first to execute such a project.
56. Ibid., pp. 4–5.
57. Ibid., p. 14, dated 14 June 1760.
58. According to Razoux, the bourgeoisie of Nîmes included domestic servants and the poor. The only unrepresentative qualities he identifies between users of the hôtel-dieu and the general population are that users were more commonly soldiers and male.
59. Ibid., pp. 82–4, including apparent errors in addition.
60. A total of 1 326 patients remained convalescent at the end of the month of entry and are here carried over into other categories or omitted. Ibid., pp. 80–256.
61. See below, pp. 85–6.
62. Peuchet, 1805, p. 272.
63. Riley, 1985, p. 43.
64. On this see especially Desaive *et al.*, 1972; Hannaway, 1972, pp. 257–73; Peter, 1971, pp. 13–38. In Desaive *et al.*, which deals only with Brittany, it is announced that studies on other parts of the archival collection will be forthcoming. The society and the Paris Faculty of Physicians agreed on the utility of such an investigation, as is evident from the faculty's endorsement in 1772 of Le Brun's proposal for a national network of medical observers who could foresee and forestall some epidemics. But the faculty was jealous of the society's privilege to execute this design.

65. Meyer, 1972, pp. 11–12. Also Hannaway, 1972, pp. 257–73; and, for a full statement of the objectives and scope of the society and its publications, see the society's *Histoire*, 1776, I, pp. viii–xxxix.
66. 1778. Also Simon, 1854, on Lépecq de La Clôture.
67. Foucault, 1973, p. 31.
68. Black, 1788, p. 37. Also Black, 1781, especially pp. 119–20; Black, 1789 (which is the second edition of Black, 1788).
69. Black, 1788, pp. 415–27.
70. Moivre, 1776 (first published 1718), pp. xiii–iv.
71. Falconer, 1781.
72. Ibid., p. 3.
73. Ibid., p. 9; Nugent, ed. (Montesquieu), 1949, p. 224, n. citing the seventeenth-century traveller Tavernier.
74. Glacken, 1967, pp. viii, 12, 581–7, and 620.
75. Magalhães, 1783 (first published 1777); Landriani, 1792 (first published 1775); Watermann, 1968, pp. 293–319, especially pp. 293–6 and 302–4.
76. E.g., Nicolas, 1786; Baumes, 1789, p. 13; and Chaptal [de Chanteloup], 1783, pp. 5–9.
77. Day, [1784], pp. 27–9.
78. W. Wright, ed. (Ramazzini), 1964 reprint, p. 7.
79. Menuret de Chambaud, 1797, p. 100. This passage is also one of the epigraphs for this chapter.

3 EPIDEMIOLOGICAL AND ENVIRONMENTAL SURVEILLANCE: COUNTING AND MEASURING PATHOGENIC SIGNS

1. Locke, 1705, p. 1 919.
2. These quotations are drawn from Hull's reprint of the fifth edition of 1676 in Hull, ed. (Petty (and Graunt)), 1963–4 reprint, II, pp. 350–1. These ideas were also present in the first edition of 1662.
3. Petty, 1755 (first published 1699), p. 40.
4. Winslow, 1943, pp. 167–8.
5. Petty 1755 (first published 1699), p. 49.
6. The trend was toward assuming a causal rather than an associative relationship. E.g., Foucault, 1973, pp. 28–9.
7. Wolff, ed. (Hume), 1969, pp. 92, 58, respectively.
8. Royston, 1970, pp. 173–81.
9. E.g., both Rutty, 1770, p. ii, and Hillary, 1766 (first published

1759), in his title, described the relationship as concomitant but also suggested a stronger, causal sense.

10. Hillary, 1811 (first published 1759), p. ii.
11. Cheyne, 1725 (first published 1724), p. xvi. In 1734 Joseph Rogers praised Cheyne as a great reasoner in 'Mathematic Knowledge', meaning, it seems, someone who reasoned from observed data. Rogers, 1734, p. xxxix.
12. See Underwood, 1950, pp. 265–74. Also Wolff, 1738 (first published 1713–15), where the Dutch translator, the physician Joan Christofel van Sprogel, asserts the usefulness of Wolff's general mathematics textbook for the physician. Gilibert, 1772, I, pp. 112–18, endorsed mathematics as an aid to medicine, but discussed chiefly its uses in logic and the understanding of form.
13. Buffon, 1749–88.
14. Fischer, 1965 reprint, II, p. 35.
15. Manley, 1959, p. 415. Also Muller, 1972, pp. 90–134; Locke, 1705, pp. 1920–37.
16. Riley, 1985, pp. 41–7.
17. Ibid., p. 42.
18. Dewhurst, 1963, p. 301.
19. Bing, 1928, pp. 249–52; Waring, 1964, I, pp. 254–60. Lining's successors, Lionel Chalmers and David Ramsay, continued his meteorological observations. See Chalmers, 1776; Ramsay, 1796; and Milligen, 1770, for an analysis of acute fevers using Lining's observations.
20. See Hales, 1731; Allan and Schofield, 1980, p. 32. Also Rogers, 1734, pp. 189–312.
21. Lining, 1742–3, p. 492. The passage concludes: 'and therefore must proceed from some general Cause operating uniformly in the returning different Seasons'.
22. Ibid., p. 493.
23. Ibid., p. 507.
24. Ibid., p. 509.
25. Lining, 1744–5, pp. 318–30.
26. Ibid., p. 319.
27. Ibid., p. 328.
28. Smyth, ed. (Stark), 1788, pp. 169–82.
29. Hillary, 1740 (first published 1735), p. 72.
30. Raulin, 1752, p. viii.
31. Ibid., p. 2.
32. Ibid., pp. 9, 15–30. Also Raulin, 1754, pp. 327–410.
33. Raulin, 1752, pp. 123–61.
34. Raulin, 1754, pp. 327–410.
35. Short, 1750, pp. 67, 167.

36. Ibid., p. 169.
37. Süssmilch, 1761–2, e.g., I, Chapter 1.
38. Millar, 1770, p. 1.

4 EPIDEMIOLOGICAL AND ENVIRONMENTAL SURVEILLANCE: REASONING ABOUT ENVIRONMENTAL PATHOGENS

1. Nugent, ed. (Montesquieu), 1949, pp. 222–3.
2. See the previous chapter.
3. As Short put it (Short, 1750, p. 84), registers of christenings and burials 'inform us which of the several Modes of Practice in Physic have been most useful'.
4. Ibid., pp. 437–43.
5. Coleman, 1982, p. 124, shows that this remained so in the early nineteenth century when 'mathematical reasoning. . .was largely confined to the computation and comparison of averages and to argumentative exploitation of simple propositions'.
6. Short, 1750, p. 81.
7. Greenwood, 1948, p. 53.
8. [Arbuthnot], 1692.
9. See Sheynin, 1970, pp. 231–9.
10. Ibid.
11. Black, 1781 (first published earlier the same year), pp. 119–20.
12. King, 1976, pp. 174–90, especially pp. 178ff.
13. Rosen, 1958, p. 106.
14. Ferré, 1968, I, p. 670.
15. Ibid.
16. Pearson, 1795, p. iv.
17. Nugent, ed. (Montesquieu), 1949, pp. 222–3.
18. Falconer, 1781, p. 3.
19. As Mary B. Hesse has shown in an argument that analogies have some value as tools of scientific logic, analogy and mathematical proportion historically 'have often been thought to be closely connected'. Hesse, 1966, p. 64.
20. For an example of this form of reasoning, as well as this specific instance of it, see Arbuthnot, 1733.
21. Huygens, 1888–1950, VI, pp. 530–2.
22. Benjamin Rush and Noah Webster are exceptions to this generalisation, in that they allowed for deferred effects.
23. Clifton, 1731, p. 22.
24. As may be seen, for example, in [Consbruch], 1793.
25. Locke, 1705, p. 1919.

26. Browne, 1972 reprint (first published 1646), pp. 208–21.
27. Bontekoe, 1683. Bontekoe was concerned to reassure the Elector Frederick William, who was nearing the age of sixty-three. In 1683 the Elector named Bontekoe professor at Frankfurt an der Oder.
28. Millar, 1779, p. 15. Petty had proposed, but not apparently executed, a similar test: compare the experience of 100 patients consulting physicians with 100 not. Also Tröhler, 1978, especially pp. 93–197, for more detail on a group Tröhler terms the 'arithmetic observationists'.
29. Millar, 1779, pp. 207–8; Tröhler, 1978, pp. 58ff.
30. Millar, 1770, p. 12. Also Tröhler, 1978, pp. 127ff. on the reservations of Robert Robertson and John Clark.
31. Black, 1788, p. 37. Also idem, 1781 (first published earlier the same year); idem, 1782; idem, 1789.
32. Black, 1788, pp. 73–4. Also Heberden, 1796, pp. 279–84. Heberden (the elder) sought to test the proposition that bracing cold is generally healthy, and warm weather generally causes putrid diseases, by comparing mortality in London during the cold spell of January 1795 and the warm spell of January 1796. He found the environment–disease association more complex that this simple relation to temperature. But he did not doubt it. Heberden (the younger), 1801, pp. 56–7, argued against the correlation of putrefaction with wetness and against some other conventional environmentalist assumptions, also without doubting the theory in general.

5 AVOIDANCE AND PREVENTION OF EPIDEMICS

1. Respectively, Baumes, 1789, p. 137; *Encyclopédie méthodique: médecine*, XIII, p. 278.
2. Caldwell, 1802, p. 45.
3. The quotation is from Banau and Turben, 1786, p. 21.
4. Baumes, 1789, p. 79.
5. Huxham, 1759–67, II, p. x.
6. Baumes, 1789, p. 7.
7. One can find some hints of hope in earlier drainage proposals. For instance, da Vinci suggested that rivers be diverted to carry eroded soil into marshes and eventually to purify the air around those marshes. Glacken, 1967, p. 465. But far more commonly drainage was justified as a means of improving agriculture. In

Italy and elsewhere it was often funded by private investors who expected to sell off the reclaimed land for profit. See ibid., pp. 476–7, 484, 488–9; Dienne, 1891, *passim*, and, it should be noted, still employing a miasmatic theory of disease propagation; Cole, 1939, I, p. 79, II, pp. 541–2; Harris, 1954–8, III, pp. 318–19.

8. *Journal oeconomique*, 1762, p. 32. Also Thouvenel, 1797–8, IV, pp. 3–48.
9. Baumes, 1789, pp. 17–18. Also Chaptal [de Chanteloup], 1783, p. 4 and *passim*.
10. Colden, 1814b, pp. 313ff (written in 1743).
11. Rush, 1786, pp. 207, 209.
12. Ibid., pp. 207–8.
13. Ibid., pp. 208–9.
14. Currie, 1799, pp. 127–42.
15. Ibid., pp. 141–2, for some other preventive measures. On the same point see T. Wright, 1799, pp. 243–6.
16. Short, 1750, p. 68; Short, 1767, pp. 35–6.
17. Muret, 1766.
18. Price, 1774, pp. 96–8. Also Lesky, ed. (Frank), 1976, pp. 177–9.
19. See [La Maillardière], 1782, especially pp. 47–50 on sources, pp. 50–80 for a geographical survey of swampy regions. Also Baumes, 1789, pp. 138–9.
20. [La Maillardière], 1782, p. 81.
21. Ibid., pp. 160–252.
22. Rawlinson, 1954–58, IV, p. 504; Cipolla, 1976, pp. 32–3.
23. Haygarth, 1778, pp. 131–4, the quote from p. 131.
24. Lesky, ed. (Frank), 1976, p. 183, which case may also be found in G. Clark, ed. (Temple), 1972, p. 80.
25. On the earlier period see Fischer, 1965 reprint, I, pp. 69–74 and *passim*.
26. Lesky, ed. (Frank), 1976, p. 184.
27. Ibid., pp. 185, 189; and, more generally, the *Archiv der medizinischen Polizey und der gemeinnützigen Arzneikunde* ed. J. C. F. Scherf from 1783–7 and its successor, 1789–99.
28. Lesky, ed. (Frank), 1976, pp. 187ff.
29. Ibid., p. ix.
30. Gilibert, 1772, III, pp. 18ff., 28. Also Michel du Tennetar, 1778, especially pp. 28–9.
31. E.g Bertholon, 1786, pp. 9–77.
32. Anon., 1782; Tournon, 1789; Bertholon, 1786, pp. 90–101. Also on the idea of medical police in Britain, Borthwick, 1784.
33. Quoted by W. Wright, ed. (Ramazzini), 1964, p. 153.
34. P. 181.
35. This association provided the Dutch physician A. P. Nahuys with material for a 1770 thesis on the healthy properties of fresh air.

Deursen, 1975, p. 68. See also Frank's ideas in Lesky, ed. (Frank), 1976, *passim*, e.g. pp. 193ff.; Smyth, 1796; [Thiroux d'Arconville], 1766, the preface; Sauvages [de la Croix], 1754, for a succinct version of eighteenth-century ideas about chemical and pneumatic means to impede putrefaction.

36. Webster, 1970 (first published 1799), II, pp. 222–3, 225. On Webster see Rosen, 1965, pp. 97–114. To Rush, 1786, p. 212, nature had even given the dung of domestic animals 'a power of destroying the effects of marsh exhalations, and of preventing fever'.
37. [Swift], 1748.
38. Webster, 1970 (first published 1799), II, p. 225.
39. Michel du Tennetar, 1778.
40. Pringle, 1749–50, pp. 480–8, 525–34, 550–8; Guyton [de] Morveau, 1801, pp. 137–76; Wasserberg, 1772, *passim*, and especially Thiroux d'Arconville, 1766, for her numerous experiments.
41. Beardsley, 1785, pp. 542–3.
42. Pringle, 1810 (first published 1752), pp. xxxiv, 74–5.
43. Ibid., p. 91. The Parisian medical topographer Menuret de Chambaud also was introduced to the field through work in military hospitals. Menuret de Chambaud, 1786, pp. 7–8.
44. Banau and Turben, 1786, p. 12.
45. Pringle, 1753, pp. 42–54. Also Singer, 1950, pp. 229–61.
46. Pringle, 1753, p. 42. Ackerknecht, 1965, p. 35, mentions five other similar incidents of typhus transmitted at court from accused to accusers. Day, [1784], pp. 2–3, added to this horror the problem of prisons so unhealthy that people accused of minor offences died before coming to trial.
47. Moheau, 1778, pt. 2, pp. 147–8; Daquin, 1787, p. 75; Devèze, 1794, pp. 38, 40, 138; Voigt, 1939, pp. 83–4. Devèze argued that burials in proximity to inhabited areas corrupt both the air and the water of wells.
48. Petty, 1755 (first published 1699), pp. 19–20.
49. Van den Bosch, 1778, pp. 361–2. Also Michel du Tennetar, 1778, pp. 22ff.
50. Roekel, 1940, pp. 839–41.
51. Bergh, 1945, p. 73.
52. Etlin, 1978, pp. 13, 66, and *passim*; Porée, 1744. Foizil and Ariès both trace intensified objections in Paris to a 1737–8 inquiry organised by the parlement of Paris. However, the results of the inquiry were not made public.
53. Haguenot, 1769. Also Piattoli, 1824 (first published 1774).
54. W. Wright, ed. (Ramazzini), 1964, pp. 151, 153.
55. [Lewis], 1721, pp. 7–35. Lewis attributed the transmission of

disease to effluvia communicated by the living (via insensible perspiration and other means) and the dead. Ibid., pp. 56, 50 (note the errors in pagination).

56. Etlin, 1978; Foisil, 1974, pp. 317ff.; Ariès, 1981, pp. 475–516. Also Tamason, 1980, pp. 15–33, on popular resistance in Lille in 1779 to cemetery relocation.
57. Rawlinson, 1954–8, IV, p. 505.
58. Lesky, ed. (Frank), 1976, p. 179.
59. E.g., Thouret, 1789; McManners, 1981, p. 43.
60. Brockington, 1966, pp. 21–2; Jones and Falkus, 1979, p. 197 and *passim.*
61. Jones and Falkus, 1979, p. 197. Ibid., pp. 212–13, detect some examples of urban improvements from the late seventeenth century, but find that the movement was concentrated after 1735.
62. [La Maillardière], 1782, p. 68.
63. Mossel, 1753, including, in the copy I examined at the Utrecht Life Insurance Company Library, Utrecht, India Council resolutions of 4 and 17 September 1753, implementing Mossel's proposals.
64. Razzell, 1965, p. 330; Hawkins, 1973 (first published 1829), p. 5; Liebel, 1965, p. 99; Payne, 1976, pp. 128–9; Glacken, 1967, pp. 487–8, 657–9.
65. Lesky, ed. (Frank), 1976, p. 179.
66. Bourde, 1967, III, p. 1 447.
67. Ibid., p. 1 448. for the quote, pp. 1 449–65, and I, pp. 532–6. And Bourde acknowledges an improvement in the salubrity of drained areas (III, p. 1 452.).
68. Anon., n.d.; Cadet de Vaux, 1784; Fournier-Choisy, 1775, especially pp. 16–18.
69. E.g., Price, 1774, pp. 96–8; [La Maillardière], 1782, *passim.* Also Baker, 1975, pp. 68–9, on Condorcet's use of mortality data to show the undesirability of building one of the Picardy canals in a marshy region.
70. That case was made by numerous writers, among them Frank, in Lesky, ed. (Frank), 1976, p. 179; Hawkins, 1973 (first published 1829), p. 203; Webster, 1970 (first published 1799), II, pp. 225–9.
71. Riley, 1985, pp. 49–50 and 134–5.
72. E.g., Earle, 1979, p. 122.
73. Lining, 1753, p. 284. Also Caldwell, 1802, pp. 13–17 and *passim.* Such ideas have a lengthy history, on which see Glacken, 1967.
74. Rush, 1786, pp. 206–12; Currie, 1972, pp. 79–80. Currie, who was eager to promote immigration, held that most of the difference had already disappeared, especially in the northern states. Ibid., pp. 398, 403. Also T. Wright, 1799, pp. 243–6, urging the clearance of forests as a method of evaporating swamps.

75. Jones and Falkus, 1979, pp. 205, 217; Perrot, 1975, II, pp. 565–7, on the profitability of relocating cemeteries in Caen.
76. Colden, 1814b, pp. 310–30; *De maandelijkse nederlandsche mercurius*, 1759, pp. 111–2; ibid., 1760, pp. 106–8; ibid., 1763, pp. 145–7; Bibliothèque nationale, Paris, Joly de Fleury papers, 1078, Projet sur le nettoyement des puits; and Chaptal [de Chanteloup], 1783, p. 22.
77. Pringle, 1753, p. 43.
78. Ibid., pp. 46–52.
79. Cited by Sand, 1952, p. 120. Also Morse and Rentmeester, 1981, pp. 63–4, 'Death Caused by Fermenting Manure', for a present-day counterpart and its explanation.
80. Pringle, 1753, p. 52.
81. Also Claude Léopold Gennété, on whose ideas see Gennété, 1767.
82. Hales, 1754, pp. 115–16. Also idem, 1758; Clark-Kennedy, 1965 reprint, especially pp. 195–207; Allan and Schofield, 1980, pp. 82–90; Gradish 1980, pp. 123–4.
83. Currie, 1799, p. 137.
84. J[aucourt], 1765, pp. 767–8; Formey, 1765, pp. 27–8; *Journal encyclopédique*, e.g., 1762, pp. 25–38, 546–7. Also Gennété, 1767.
85. Clark-Kennedy, 1965 reprint, pp. 152–3, 162–3.
86. Lloyd, ed., 1965, p. 182; Lloyd and Coulter, 1961, pp. 72–4.
87. Great Britain, 1774, pp. 1 391–4.
88. See Goldin, 1976, pp. 512–35; Le Roy, 1793, pp. 348–50; Etlin, 1978, pp. 177–81.
89. The list of gifts received during the previous year in TAPs, (1793), III, p. 351.
90. Clark-Kennedy, 1965 reprint, pp. 168–9, 169, n. Also Lloyd and Coulter, 1961, III, pp. 72–4; Lloyd, ed., 1965, pp. 181–9.
91. Good, 1795, pp. 121–3.
92. Lind, 1779 (first published 1757), pp. 313–4.
93. Fischer, 1965 reprint, II, pp. 228–9; Van den Bosch, 1778, p. 362, n. E.
94. Ockerse, 1792, pp. 43 and *passim*, indicates some cities where cemeteries were established before 1795.
95. Roekel, 1940, pp. 840–1.
96. Anon., 1783. Also Piattoli, 1824 (first published 1774), pp. 73, 79–82.
97. Thouret, 1789; for the quote, Ragon, 1983, p. 62. Also Etlin, 1978, pp. 72–95 and *passim*; Hannaway and Hannaway, 1977, pp. 181–92; Foizil, 1974, pp. 303–30; Ariès, 1981, pp. 498–9; McManners, 1981, pp. 303–19.
98. Cambry, 1799.
99. Ariès, 1981. pp. 483–6 (quote from p. 486).
100. Ibid., pp. 491, 495–6.
101. Ibid., especially pp. 318ff.

102. Ibid., pp. 68, 92 (quote from p. 92).
103. Corbin, 1982, pp. ii and *passim*.
104. E. L. Jones, 1981, pp. 127–49. See also Kunitz, 1983, pp. 353–5; Perrot, 1975, I, pp. 11–2 and *passim*; Huard, 1958, p. 4 483.

6 MEDICAL EFFECTS OF ENVIRONMENTAL ENGINEERING

1. Bisset, 1762, preface.
2. White, 1782, p. 43.
3. Also Baumes, 1789, pp. 141–3, on drainage.
4. But there were areas of exception (e.g., apparently, Anjou, on which see Lebrun, 1971, especially pp. 261–9, 491–2).
5. McKeown, 1976, pp. 65–71.
6. Kunitz, 1983, pp. 349–64.
7. Perrenoud, 1979, I, p. 423; Puranen, 1984, pp. 123, 125 (tuberculosis mortality in Sweden rose during 1750–1830 from 7 to 8 per cent of all deaths to over 11 per cent); Lee, 1980, pp. 261–2.
8. Armengaud, 1973, p. 33; Reinhard, *et al.*, 1968, pp. 680–1.
9. Riley, 1985, pp. 76–9, 82.
10. See the sources cited in note 6 in the Introduction, especially Wrigley and Schofield, 1981; Bruneel, 1977, I, p. 350; Chambers, 1957, p. 33; Perrenoud, 1979; Hofsten and Lundström, 1976, especially p. 16.
11. McKeown and Brown, 1955, pp. 119–41. Also McKeown, 1976; McKeown, 1983.
12. Razzell, 1977; Razzell, 1965; Bynum, 1980. pp. 247–8.
13. McKeown, 1976, pp. 12, 108.
14. Miller, 1962; Lee, 1980, pp. 247–8.
15. McKeown, 1976, pp. 128–42; Flinn, 1981, pp. 95–7, 101.
16. Turner, 1982, p. 506 believes so; but Overton, 1984, pp. 244–57, has serious doubts.
17. Lee, 1980, pp. 244–68.
18. Tilly, 1971, pp. 37–40.
19. Anon., 1983, p. 506. Also Livi-Bacci, 1983, pp. 293–8. An individual infected with tuberculosis will more probably develop an active case if poorly nourished, but nutrition does not play a role in infection, which is air-borne.
20. Carmichael, 1983, pp. 249, 264 respectively. Also Dobson, 1980, pp. 385–6, hypothesising that a barrier was passed. Below it, a host of diseases contributed collectively to debilitation and short life expectations; above it, diseases no longer assisted one another.
21. Deane, 1965, pp. 6–7, *vis-à-vis* England and Wales in the middle

of the eighteenth century. *Per capita* income in the Dutch Republic may still have exceeded that in England.

22. Flinn, 1974, p. 295. Also Wrigley and Schofield, 1981, pp. 450–1; Flinn, 1981, pp. 47–51; the work of Pierre Goubert, e.g., Goubert, 1970, pp. 23–4 and *passim.*
23. Flinn, 1974, p. 315.
24. Ibid., p. 316.
25. E. L. Jones, 1978, p. 114.
26. Anderson, 1981, pp. 337–55.
27. McKeown, 1976, pp. 73–90, especially pp. 89–90.
28. Kunitz, 1983, pp. 349–64.
29. McKeown and Brown, 1955, p. 141.
30. In later work McKeown (1976, 1978) argues that public health improvements – by which he has in mind specific measures such as the provision of safe drinking water – occurred only in the late nineteenth century. He does not deal with the improvements treated here except in relation to typhus.
31. Dupâquier, 1978, p. 240.
32. Meyer, 1972, p. 13.
33. Flinn, 1981, pp. 89–101.
34. McManners, 1981, pp. 52–3.
35. Dupâquier, 1979, p. 34.
36. McKeown, 1976, p. 107, argues that James Lind showed in 1786 that too small doses had customarily been given.
37. Newman, 1965, p. 1.
38. Ibid., pp. 13–14.
39. Ibid., p. 77.
40. Smith, 1981, p. 123.
41. Bruce-Chwatt and de Zulueta, 1980, p. 69.
42. McKeown, 1976, p. 16.
43. Hirsch, 1883–6, I, pp. 215–19. Also Ackerknecht, 1965, pp. 90–2; Bruce-Chwatt and de Zulueta, 1980, pp. 2, 134–5, and *passim.* Voigt, 1939, p. 84, found malaria a disease of major importance in eighteenth-century Germany.
44. McKeown, 1976, p. 113.
45. Horsfall, 1955, pp. 44–308 *passim*, especially pp. 61, 93.
46. Bruce-Chwatt and de Zulueta, 1980, pp. 134–5. Also McManners, 1981, pp. 6, 23, on malaria as a leading cause of death in France.
47. Chambers, 1972, p. 98.
48. Anning, 1984, p. 421 and n., suggesting that ague covers a variety of fevers, including malaria.
49. J. Woodward, 1974, p. 37. Also MacArthur, 1951, pp. 76, 79; Lind, 1777 (first published 1768), p. 302; and Bibliothèque nationale, Paris, Joly de Fleury papers, 1079, 30.

50. Hawkins, 1973 (first published 1829), pp. 189, 196.
51. McNeill, 1976, pp. 218–19.
52. Bruce-Chwatt and de Zulueta, 1980, p. 5.
53. Ackerknecht, 1965, pp. 91, 94. Also idem, 1945, pp. 62–130, for an extended discussion of factors associated with the disappearance of malaria in the Upper Mississippi Valley before the advent of an eradication programme.
54. Bruce-Chwatt and de Zulueta, 1980, p. 112.
55. Hackett, 1952, p. 43.
56. Dobson, 1980, pp. 357–89.
57. Ibid., p. 382.
58. Ibid., p. 386.
59. Ibid., p. 384 and n. 6.
60. Bruce-Chwatt and de Zulueta, 1980, p. 4.
61. Riley, 1980, p. 17.
62. Bruce-Chwatt and de Zulueta, 1980, p. 8. Despite recurrent efforts, drainage of the Pontine marshes was not made fully effective until the 1930s.
63. Russell, 1959, pp. 418–9.
64. Bourde, 1967, III, p. 1 452.
65. Archives nationales, Paris, H[1] 1 488.
66. Ibid., H[1] 1 488–98, contain information on numerous disputes during the 1770s and 1780s over this issue.
67. Rutman and Rutman, 1976, p. 50, also apply the modern conception of malaria as a debilitating disease to explain high mortality in Virginia in the late seventeenth and early eighteenth century. According to this source (p. 51), the northern boundary of malaria in the United States shifted southward during the eighteenth century.
68. Dobson, 1980, p. 385.
69. Greenbaum, 1976, p. 902. Also Jones and Sonenscher, 1983, 172–214; Foucault *et al.*, 1976, especially pp. 55–69.
70. Greenbaum, 1974, pp. 122–40; Percival, 1776a, pp. 171–86.
71. Peuchet, 1805, p. 256.
72. See McKeown, 1976, p. 114, on droplet removal.
73. Hawkins, 1973, (first published 1829), pp. 79, 196.
74. McKeown, 1976, p. 106.
75. Ibid., p. 114.
76. Riley, 1981, p. 653, n. 3.
77. Klein and Engerman, 1979, p. 271.
78. Clark-Kennedy, 1965 reprint, pp. 161–3.
79. Gradish, 1980, p. 124.
80. Ibid., p. 120.
81. Ibid., pp. 201, 208.
82. Mathias, 1975, p. 79; Allan and Schofield, 1980, p. 161, n. 29.

83. Hawkins, 1973 (first published 1829), p. 189.
84. Busvine, 1976, pp. 188, 190–1, 193.
85. Greenberg, 1965, p. 93. Also West, 1951, pp. 117–8 and *passim.*
86. Rosen, 1958, p. 183.
87. Shryock, 1936, pp. 78–106.

7 CONCLUSION

1. Peter, 1972, p. 139.
2. E.g., Bigel, an VII (1798–9); Tourtelle, 1819; Borthwick, 1784; and Audin-Rouvière, an II (1793–4).
3. Hallé, 1787, p. 492. On Hallé and the Paris school see Coleman, 1982, pp. 4–24.
4. Ramel, 1785, pp. 353–90. Also Moreau de la Sarth, [1800?].
5. Rush, 1794; Carey, 1793a; Carey, 1793b; Rush, 1793–1809 (first published various dates), IV, pp. 3–258, and V, the entire volume; Currie, 1798; Nassy, 1793; Devèze, 1794; Davidge, 1798; Powell, 1949; Winslow, 1943, pp. 196–235; Winslow *et al.*, 1952, pp. 31–44. Also T. Woodward, 1980, pp. 115–31; Duffy, 1971 reprint, pp. 138–63.
6. See Ackerknecht, 1965, pp. 50–9.
7. Goodyear, 1978, p. 5.
8. This is reminiscent of the environmentalist explanation of an epidemic that began at Wadham College, Oxford, many years earlier. In that instance the putrefaction of some cabbages was believed to have been the cause. Rogers, 1734, p. 41.
9. In addition to the sources cited in note 5 above, see La Roche, 1855, I, pp. 73–4; Helmuth, 1794, p. 8; and Lining, 1799 (the publication in Philadelphia of his description of the Charleston epidemic of 1748).
10. By 1803 Rush rejected any role for contagion. Rush, 1803, pp. 136, 147.
11. Also Devèze, 1794, p. 16, who arrived in Philadelphia on the eve of the epidemic: 'the first cause of this scourge is the same which produces almost all other diseases, the alteration of the atmospheric air'.
12. Carey, 1793a, pointed out, however, that earlier authors on the disease had not specified putrid vegetable matter as a source.
13. Rush, 1803, pp. 135–50.
14. Ibid., p. 136.
15. Carey, 1793b, pp. 21–2, detailing recommendations offered by the College of Physicians and the mayor, Matthew Clarkson.
16. Ackerknecht, 1948, pp. 567, 587, 590–1; Rosenberg, 1962, pp. 19–20.

17. Shryock, 1936, pp. 137–8; Cassedy, 1969a, pp. 292–4.
18. Rush, 1794, pp. 270ff.; idem, 1793–1809, IV, pp. 183–258. Also Holmes, 1966, pp. 246–63.
19. Bryce, 1796, reporting his experience aboard an East Indiaman in 1792.
20. Webster, 1970 (first published 1799), I, p. vii; Webster, 1979 (first published 1797–8), *passim*. Jordonova, 1979, pp. 119–46, discusses other non-medical writers on environmentalist topics.
21. Webster, 1970 (first published 1799), II, p. 10.
22. Ibid., I, p. 288.
23. The idea that smallpox did not fit the pattern of other diseases seems to derive in part from the observations of William Douglass, an environmentalist physician who practiced in Boston, and from Thomas Percival's conclusions after studying three smallpox epidemics. In the early 1750s Douglass reported that, in his experience, smallpox death rates were little related to season, climate, or geography. Cassedy, 1969b, pp. 198–9; Weaver, 1917–21, pp. 230–2; Percival, 1776a, pp. 95–6.
24. As remarked by T. Woodward, 1980, p. 119.
25. The plans announced in 1972 in Desaive *et al.* and Meyer to provide extended analyses of these data seem not to have been fulfilled.
26. Foucault, 1973, p. 31. In 1800 the statistician J. A. Mourgue repeated the hope that additional, and especially more precise, information would clarify understanding of the influence of environmental factors on fertility and mortality. Mourgue, [1800], pp. 1–3. Also Bouffey, an VII (1798–9) – 1813, I, pp. 6–8, 43, and *passim*. The problem of excessive data was not merely an eighteenth-century issue. McGlashan, ed., 1972, p. 4, explains that the field of medical geography was slow to develop in its twentieth-century revival because of inadequate analytical tools for interpreting too abundant data, a problem overcome by statistical geography.
27. Carey, 1793b, at the end.
28. King, 1963a, pp. 90–134.
29. Rush, 1794, pp. 108–9.
30. La Roche, 1855, I, pp. 66–8.
31. This notwithstanding temporary and mild seizures reported by both Rush and Devèze.
32. Winslow, 1943, p. 175.
33. Ibid., p. x.
34. Andersen, 1979, p. 14.
35. See the sources cited in the Introduction, note 8.

Bibliography

ABBREVIATIONS

AMPR	*American Medical and Philosophical Register*
BHM	*Bulletin of the History of Medicine*
BMB	*British Medical Bulletin*
CS	*Ciba Symposia*
DHS	*Dix-Huitième Siècle*
JIH	*Journal of Interdisciplinary History*
JHM	*Journal of the History of Medicine and Allied Sciences*
MH	*Medical History*
NTG	*Nederlandsch Tijdschrift voor Geneeskunde*
PT	*Philosophical Transactions*
TAPS	*Transactions of the American Philosophical Society*

MANUSCRIPT SOURCES

Archives nationales, Paris, H[1] 1 488–98, *Partage des biens communaux; defrichements et desséchements de marais...1603–1790.*

Bibliothèque nationale, Paris, *Joly de Fleury Papers, 1 078–80*, various memoirs on public health measures and population issues.

PRINTED SOURCES

Ackerknecht, Erwin H., 'Anticontagionism between 1821 and 1867', BHM, XXII (September–October 1948), 562–93.

——'The Development of Our Knowledge of Malaria', CS, VII (April–May 1945), 38–50.

——*History and Geography of the Most Important Diseases*, New York, 1965.

——'Hygiene in France, 1815–1848', BHM, XXII (March–April 1948), 117–55.

——Malaria in the Upper Mississippi Valley, 1760–1900*, Baltimore, 1945.
——*Medicine at the Paris Hospital, 1794–1848*, Baltimore, 1967.

Aitken, George A., *The Life and Works of John Arbuthnot*, Oxford, 1892.

[Alembert, Jean le Rond d'], 'Emanations', *Encyclopédie, ou dictionnaire raisonné des sciences*, V, 1755, 545–6.

Allan, D. G. C. and R. E. Schofield, *Stephen Hales: Scientist and Philanthropist*, London, 1980.

Andersen, Otto, 'The Development of Danish Mortality, 1735–1850', *Scandinavian Population Studies*, V (1979), 9–21.

Anderson J. L., 'History and Climate: Some Economic Models', in T. M. L. Wigley, M. J. Ingram, and G. Farmer (eds), *Climate and History: Studies in Past Climates and Their Impact on Man*, Cambridge, 1981, 337–55.

Anning, S. T., 'A Medical Case Book: Leeds, 1781–84', MH, XXVIII (October 1984), 420–31.

Anon., *Eenige algemeene regelen tot de bewaring der gezondheid en voorkoming van ziekten onder de bewoonders der geïnundeerde landen*, n.p., n.d.

——*Réflexions...sur la nature de la constitution de cette année, & le traitment des maladies qu'elle a occasionnées* [Paris, 1781].

——*Vues sur la propreté des rues de Paris*, n.p., 1782.

——*Recueil de pièces concernant les exhumations faites dans l'enceinte de l'Eglise de Saint Eloy de la ville de Dunkerque*, Paris, 1783.

——Parts of the the article 'Air', *Encyclopédie méthodique: médecine*, I, 1787, 568–75.

——'The Relationship of Nutrition, Disease, and Social Conditions: A Graphical Presentation', JIH, XIV (Autumn 1983), 503–6.

Arbuthnot, John, 'An Argument for Divine Providence, Taken from the Constant Regularity Observ'd in the Births of Both Sexes', PT, XXVII (1710–12), 186–90.

—— *An Essay Concerning the Effects of Air on Human Bodies*, London, 1733.

[Arbuthnot, John], 'Essay on the Usefulness of Mathematical Learning' in George A. Aitken, *The Life and Works of John Arbuthnot*, Oxford, 1892.

—— *Of the Laws of Chance, or, A Method of Calculation of the Hazards of Game*, mainly a translation of C. Huygens, *De ratiociniis in ludo aleae*, London, 1692.

Archiv der medizinischen Polizey und der gemeinnützigen Arzneikunde' (ed.) Johann Christian Friedrich Scherf, 6 vols, Leipzig, 1783–7.

Ariès, Philippe, *The Hour of Our Death*, trans. Helen Weaver, New York, 1981.

Armengaud, André, 'Population in Europe, 1700–1914', in Carlo M. Cipolla (ed), *The Fontana Economic History of Europe*, vol. 3, London, 1973.

[Astruc, Jean], *Dissertation sur l'origine des maladies épidémiques*, Montpellier, 1721.

Audin-Rouvière, [Joseph Marie], *Essai sur la topographie-physique et médicale de Paris*, [Paris], an II (1793–4).

Baillou, Guillaume de, *Epidémies et éphémérides*, trans. Prosper Yvaren, Paris, 1858.

Baker, Keith Michael, *Condorcet: From Natural Philosophy to Social Mathematics*, Chicago, 1975.

Banau, [Jean Baptiste] and [François] Turben, *Mémoire sur les épidémies du Languedoc*, Paris, 1786.

Barker, John, *An Essay on the Agreement betwixt Ancient and Modern Physicians: or a Comparison between the Practice of Hippocrates, Galen, Sydenham, and Boerhaave*, London, 1747.

Barkhuus, Arne, 'Medical Geographies', CS, VI (January 1945), 1 997–2 016.

_____ 'Medical Surveys from Hippocrates to the World Travellers', CS, VI (January 1945), 1986–96.

Bates, Donald George, *Thomas Sydenham: The Development of His Thought, 1666–1676*, unpublished Ph.D. dissertation, Johns Hopkins University, 1975.

Baumes, [J. B. T.], *Mémoire qui a remporté le prix, en 1789, au jugement de la Société Royale de Médecine de Paris, sur la question proposée en ces termes: Déterminer, par l'observation, quelles sont les maladies qui résultent des émanations des eaux stagnantes*, Nîmes, 1789.

Beardsley, Ebenezer, 'Remarks on the Effects of Stagnant Air', *Memoirs of the American Academy of Arts and Sciences*, I (1785), 542–3.

Beattie, Lester M., *John Arbuthnot, Mathematician and Satirist*, Cambridge, Mass., 1935.

Behrends, Johann Adolph, *Der Einwohner in Frankfurt am Mayn in Absicht auf seine Fruchtbarkeit, Mortalität und Gesundheit geschildert*, Frankfurt, 1771.

Bent, William, *A Meteorological Journal of the Year 1795*, London, 1796.

Bergh, Adrianus Johannes van den, *Utrechtsche hygiënische vraagstukken; historisch beschouwd*, Utrecht, 1945.

Bertholon, Pierre, *De la salubrité de l'air des villes, et en particulier des moyens de la procurer*, Montpellier, 1786.

[Bertin, Antoine], *Des moyens de conserver la santé des blancs et des négres, aux Antilles*, Santo Domingo, 1768.

Bigel, *Topographie médicale de Mâcon*, Mâcon, an VII (1798–9).

Bing, Franklin C., 'John Lining: An Early American Scientist', *Scientific Monthly*, XXVI (March 1928), 249–52.

Bisset, Charles, *An Essay on the Medical Constitution of Great Britain*, London, 1762.

_____ *Medical Essays and Observations*, Newcastle upon Tyne, 1766.

Black, William, *An Arithmetical and Medical Analysis of the Diseases and Mortality of the Human Species*, 2nd edn, London, 1789.

——*A Comparative View of the Mortality of the Human Species*, London, 1788.

——*An Historical Sketch of Medicine and Surgery*, London, 1782.

——*Observations Medical and Political, on the Small Pox*, 2nd edn, London, 1781.

Blake, John B., *A Short Title Catalogue of Eighteenth Century Printed Books in the National Library of Medicine*, Bethesda, Md., 1979.

Blayo, Yves, 'La mortalité en France de 1740 à 1829', *Population*, XXX (Special number of November 1975), 123–42.

Blom, Carl Magnus, 'Observationes de aëre et morbis epidemicis in Dahlekarlia svecorum, ab initio anni 1772 ad finem anni 1773', *Acta medicorum Svecicorum*, I (1783), 433–77.

Boix y Moliner, Miguel Marcelino, *Hippocrates aclarado: y sistema de Galeno impugnado*, Madrid, 1716.

Bonnet, T., 'Un fléau ancien trop méconnu: l'habitat insolubre', *Soins: Revue medicale des communautes religieuses*, XXIII (5 June 1978), 49–56.

Bontekoe, Cornelis, *Kort en vast bewijs dat 'er geen annus climactericus of moort-jaar is*, The Hague, 1683.

Borthwick, George, *The Method of Preventing and Removing the Causes of Infectious Diseases*, Cork, 1784.

Bosch, Iman Jacob van den, *Verhandelingen uitgegeeven door de Hollandsche Maatschappije der Weetenschappen . . . vervattende het antwoord op de vraage: Welken zijn de ziekten onder de menschen, die uit de natuurlijke gesteldheid van het vaderland voortvloeijen?*, Haarlem, 1778.

Bouffey, L[ouis] D[ominique] A[mable], *Recherches sur l'influence de l'air dans le développement, le caractère et le traitement des maladies*, 2 vols, Paris, an VII (1798–9)–1813.

Boulton, Richard, *Some Thoughts Concerning the Unusual Qualities of the Air*, London, 1724.

Bourde, André J., *Agronomie et agronomes en France au XVIIIe siècle*, 3 vols, Paris, 1967.

Boyle, Robert, 'General Heads for a Natural History of a Countrey, Great or Small', PT, no. 11 (April 1666), 186–9.

——*The General History of the Air*, London, 1692.

Brockington, C. Fraser, *A Short History of Public Health*, 2nd edn, London, 1966.

Browne, Thomas, *Pseudodoxia Epidemica: or, Enquiries into Commonly Presumed Truths*, Mention, 1972 reprint of 1646 edition.

Brownrigg, William, *Considerations on the Means of Preventing the Communication of Pestilential Contagion*, London, 1771.

Bruce-Chwatt, Leonard Jan, and Julian de Zulueta, *The Rise and Fall of Malaria in Europe: A Historico-epidemiological Study*, Oxford, 1980.

Brügelmann, Jan, 'Observations on the Process of Medicalisation in Germany, 1770–1830, Based on Medical Topographies', *Historical Reflections*, IX (Spring and Summer 1975), 131–49.

Bruneel, Claude, *La mortalité dans les campagnes: Le duché de Brabant aux XVIIe et XVIIIe siècles*, 2 vols, Leuven, 1977.

Bryce, James, *An Account of the Yellow Fever*, Edinburgh, 1796.

[Buffon, Georges Louis Leclerc de], *Histoire naturelle*, 20 vols, Paris 1749–88.

Burggrave, Johann Philipp, *De aere, aquis & locis urbis Francofurtanae ad Moenum commentatio*, Frankfurt, 1751.

Busvine, J. R., *Insects, Hygiene and History*, London, 1976.

Bynum, W. F., 'Health, Disease and Medical Care', in G. S. Rousseau and Roy Porter (eds), *The Ferment of Knowledge: Studies in the Historiography of Eighteenth-Century Science*, Cambridge, 1980.

Cadet de Vaux, [Antoine Alexis], *Avis sur les moyens de diminuer l'insalubrité des habitations qui ont été exposées aux inondations*, Paris, 1784.

Caldwell, Charles, *An Oration on the Causes of the Difference, in Point of Frequency and Force, Between the Endemic Diseases of the United States of America, and Those of the Countries of Europe*, Philadelphia, 1802.

Cambry,[Jacques de], *Rapport sur les sépultures*, Paris, an VII (1799).

Carey, Mathew, *Observations on Dr. Rush's Enquiry into the Origin of the Late Epidemic Fever in Philadelphia*, Philadelphia, 1793a.

_____*A Short Account of the Malignant Fever, Lately Prevalent in Philadelphia*, 2nd edn, Philadelphia, 1793b.

Carmichael, Ann G., 'Infection, Hidden Hunger, and History', JIH, XIV (Autumn 1983), 249–64.

Cartwright, Frederick F., *A Social History of Medicine*, London, 1977.

Cassedy, James H., *Demography in Early America: Beginnings of the Statistical Mind, 1600–1800*, Cambridge, Mass., 1969a.

_____'Medicine and the Rise of Statistics', in Allen G. Debus (ed), *Medicine in Seventeenth Century England*, Berkeley, 1974.

_____'Meteorology and Medicine in Colonial America: Beginnings of the Experimental Approach', JHM, XXIV (April 1969) 1969b, 193–204.

Chadwick, John and W. N. Mann (eds and trans.), *The Medical Works of Hippocrates*, Oxford, 1950.

Chalmers, Lionel, *An Account of the Weather and Diseases of South-Carolina*, 2 vols, London, 1776.

Chambers, J. D., *Population, Economy, and Society in Pre-Industrial England*, Oxford, 1972.

_____ *The Vale of Trent, 1670–1800: A Regional Study of Economic Change*, London, 1957.

Chaptal [de Chanteloup], J[ean] A[ntoine Claude], *Mémoire sur les causes de l'insalubrité des lieux voisins de nos étangs, et sur les moyens d'y remédier*, Montpellier, 1783.

Chevalier, [Jean Damien], *Lettres à M. de Jean . . . sur les maladies de St. Domingue*, Paris, 1752.

Cheyne, George, *An Essay of Health and Long Life*, 4th edn, London, 1725.

Cipolla, Carlo M., *Public Health and the Medical Profession in the Renaissance*, Cambridge, 1976.

Clark, George (ed.), *Observations upon the United Provinces of the Netherlands* (by William Temple), Oxford, 1972.

Clark, John, *Observations on the Diseases Which Prevail in Long Voyages to Hot Countries*, 2nd edn rev., 2 vols, London, 1792.

Clark-Kennedy, A. E., *Stephen Hales: An Eighteenth Century Biography*, Cambridge, 1965 reprint.

Cleghorn, George, *Observations on the Epidemical Diseases in Minorca from the Year 1744, to 1749*, 4th edn, London, 1779.

Clifton, Francis, *Tabular Observations Recommended, as the Plainest and Surest Way of Practicing and Improving Physick*, London, 1731.

Colden, Cadwallader, 'An Account of the Climate and Diseases of New York', AMPR, I (1814 reprint of 1810–11 edn) 1814a, 304–10.

——'Observations on the Fever Which Prevailed in the City of New-York in 1741 and 2, Written in 1743', AMPR, I (1814 reprint of 1810–11 edn) 1814b, 310–30.

Cole, Charles Woolsey, *Colbert and a Century of French Mercantilism*, 2 vols, New York, 1939.

Coleman, William, *Death is a Social Disease: Public Health and Political Economy in Early Industrial France*, Madison, 1982.

——'Health and Hygiene in the *Encyclopédie*: A Medical Doctrine for the Bourgeoisie', JHM, XXIX (October 1974), 399–421.

—— 'L'hygiène et l'état selon Montyon', DHS, IX (1977), 101–8.

Collin, Nicholas, 'An Essay on Those Inquiries in Natural Philosophy, Which at Present are Most Beneficial to the United States', TAPS, III (1793), iii–xxvii.

[Consbruch, Georg Wilhelm Christoph] *Medicinische Ephemeriden nebst einer medicinischen Topographie der Grafschaft Ravensberg*, Chemnitz, 1793.

Corbin, Alain, *La miasma et la jonquille: L'odorat et l'imaginaire social, XVIIIe-XIXe siècles*, Paris, 1982.

Cotte, [Louis], *Mémoires sur la météorologie*, 2 vols, Paris, 1788.

——*Traité de météorologie*, Paris, 1774.

Craig, W. S., *History of the Royal College of Physicians of Edinburgh*, Oxford, 1976.

Creighton, Charles, *A History of Epidemics in Britain*, 2 vols, Cambridge, 1891–4.

Crookshank, F[rancis] G[raham], *Epidemiological Essays*, London, 1930.

Currie, William, 'An Enquiry into the Causes of the Insalubrity of Flat and Marshy Situations', TAPS, IV (1799), 127–142.

——*An Historical Account of the Climates and Diseases of the United States*, New York, 1972 reprint.

——*Observations on the Causes and Cure of Remitting or Bilious Fevers*, Philadelphia, 1798.

Daquin, Joseph, *Topographie medicale de la ville de Chambéry et de ses environs*, Chambéry, 1787.

Davidge, John B., *A Treatise on the Autumnal Endemial Epidemick of Tropical Climates, Vulgarly Called the Yellow Fever*, Baltimore, 1798.

Day, Thomas, *Some Considerations on the Different Ways of Removing Confined and Infectious Air; and the Means Adopted, with Remarks on the Contagion in Maidstone Gaol*, Maidstone, [1784].

Dazille, [Jean Barthélemy], *Observations générales sur les maladies des climats chauds*, Paris, 1785.

Deane, Phyllis, *The First Industrial Revolution*, Cambridge, 1965.

Dedieu, Joseph, *Montesquieu et la tradition politique anglaise en France*, New York, 1970 reprint.

Deparcieux, Antoine, *Essai sur les probabilités de la durée de la vie humaine*, Paris, 1746.

Desaive, Jean-Paul *et al.*, *Médecins, climat et épidémies à la fin du XVIIIe siècle*, Paris, 1972.

Deursen, A. Th. van, 'History and Prognostication', in *Acta Historiae Neerlandicae*, VIII, 1975.

Devèze, Jean, *An Enquiry into and Observations upon the Causes and Effects of the Epidemic Disease, Which Raged in Philadelphia*, Philadelphia, 1794.

Dewhurst, Kenneth, 'The Genesis of State Medicine in Ireland', *Irish Journal of Medical Science*, no. 368 (August 1956), 365–84.

_____*John Locke, 1632–1704, Physician and Philosopher: A Medical Biography*, London, 1963.

_____*Dr. Thomas Sydenham (1624–1689): His Life and Original Writings*, Berkeley, 1966.

_____'A Review of John Locke's Research in Social and Preventive Medicine', BMH, XXXVI (July–August 1962), 317–40.

Dienne, [Louis Edouard Marie Hippolyte de], *Histoire du dessèchement des lacs et marais en France avant 1789*, Paris, 1891.

Dobson, Mary, 'Marsh Fever–The Geography of Malaria in England', *Journal of Historical Geography*, VI (1980), 357–89.

Duffy, John, *Epidemics in Colonial America*, Baton Rouge, 1971 reprint.

Dupâquier, Jacques, *La population française aux XVIIe et XVIIIe siècles*, Paris, 1979.

_____'Révolution française et révolution demographique', in Ernest Hinrichs, *et al.*, (eds), *Vom Ancien Régime zur Französischen Revolution*, Göttingen, 1978.

Duvillard [de Durand], E. E., *Analyse et tableaux de l'influence de la petite vérole sur la mortalité*, Paris, 1806.

Duyn, Nicolaas, *Aanmerkingen en aanteekeningen, van drie meer dan gemeene strenge winters*, Haarlem, 1744.

Earle, Carville V., 'Environment, Disease, and Mortality in Early

Virginia', in Thad W. Tate and David L. Ammerman (eds), *The Chesapeake in the Seventeenth Century*, Chapel Hill, 1979.

Emch-Dériaz, Antoinette Suzanne, 'Towards a Social Conception of Health in the Second Half of the Eighteenth Century: Tissot (1728–1797) and the New Preoccupation with Health and Well-Being', Ph.D. dissertation, University of Rochester, 1983.

Encyclopédie méthodique: Médecine, 13 vols, Paris, 1787–1830.

Erndtel, Christian Heinrich, *Warsavia physice illustrata, sive de aere, aquis, locis et incolis Warsaviae, eorundemque moribus et morbis tractatus*, Dresden, 1730.

Etlin, Richard Allan, 'L'air dans l'urbanisme des Lumières', DHS, IX (1977), 123–34.

——'The Cemetery and the City: Paris, 1744–1804', Ph.D. dissertation, Princeton University, 1978.

Eyler, John M., *Victorian Social Medicine: The Ideas and Methods of William Farr*, Baltimore, 1979.

——'William Farr on the Cholera: The Sanitarian's Disease Theory and the Statistician's Method', JHM, XXVIII (April 1973), 79–100.

Falconer, William, *Remarks on the Influence of Climate, Situation, Nature of Country*, London, 1781.

Favre, Robert, 'Du "medico-topographique" à Lyon en 1783', DHS, IX (1977), 151–60.

Ferré, Frederick, 'Design Argument', in Philip P. Wiener (ed.), *Dictionary of the History of Ideas*, 4 vols, New York, 1968.

Finke, Leonhard Ludwig, *Versuch einer allgemeinen medicinisch-praktischen Geographie*, 3 vols, Leipzig, 1792–5.

Fischer, Alfons, *Geschichte des deutschen Gesundheitswesens*, 2 vols, Berlin, 1965 reprint.

Flinn, Michael, *The European Demographic System, 1500–1820*, Baltimore, 1981.

——'The Population History of England, 1541–1871' [A Review], *Economic History Review*, XXXV (August 1982), 443–57.

——'The Stabilisation of Mortality in Pre-industrial Western Europe', *Journal of European Economic History*, III (Fall 1974), 285–318.

Foisil, Madeleine, 'Les attitudes devant la mort au XVIIIe siècle: sépultures et suppressions de sépultures dans le cimetière parisien des Saints-Innocents', *Revue historique*, no 510 (April-June 1974), 303–30.

Formey, Jean Henri Samuel, 'Ventilateur', in the *Encyclopédie, ou dictionnaire raisonné des sciences*, XVII, 1765, 27–8.

Foucault, Michel, *The Birth of the Clinic: An Archaeology of Medical Perception*, trans. A. M. Sheridan Smith, New York, 1973.

——*et al.*, *Les machines à guérir*, Paris, 1976.

Fournier-Choisy, *Mémoire sur les maladies épidémiques qu'occasionne ordinairement le dessèchement des marais*, Bordeaux, 1775.

Frisinger, H. Howard, *The History of Meteorology: to 1800*, New York, 1977.

Galdston, Iago, 'Social Medicine and the Epidemic Constitution', BHM, XXV (January–February 1951), 8–21.

Gelfand, Toby, *Professionalizing Modern Medicine: Paris Surgeons and Medical Science and Institutions in the 18th Century*, Westport, Conn., 1980.

Genneté, [Claude Léopold], *Purification de l'air croupissant dans les hôpitaux, les prisons & les vaisseaux de mer*, Nancy, 1767.

Geoffroy, [Etienne Louis], *L'hygieine; ou l'art de conserver la santé*, trans. de Launay, Paris, 1774.

Gesscher, David van, *Heelkunde van Hippocrates*, Amsterdam, 1790.

Gilibert, J[ean] E[mmanuel], *L'anarchie médicinale, ou la médecine considérée comme nuisible à la société*, 3 vols, Neuchâtel, 1772.

Glacken, Clarence J., *Traces on the Rhodian Shore: Nature and Culture in Western Thought from Ancient Times to the End of the Eighteenth Century*, Berkeley, 1967.

Goad, [John], *Astro-meteorologica, or Aphorisms and Discourses of the Bodies Celestial, their Natures and Influences*, London, 1686.

Goldin, Grace, 'Building a Hospital of Air: The Victorian Pavilions of St. Thomas' Hospital, London', BHM, IL (Winter 1976), 512–35.

Good, John Mason, *A Dissertation on the Diseases of Prisons and Poor-Houses*, London, 1795.

Goodyear, James D., 'The Sugar Connection: A New Perspective on the History of Yellow Fever', BHM, LII (Spring 1978), 5–21.

Goubert, Pierre, *Louis XIV and Twenty Million Frenchmen*, trans. Anne Carter, New York, 1970.

Gradish, Stephen F., *The Manning of the British Navy durirg the Seven Years' War*, London, 1980.

Grant, William, *An Essay on the Pestilential Fever of Sydenham*, London, 1775.

Graunt, John, *Natural and Political Observations made upon the Bills of Mortality*, 4th edn, Oxford, 1665.

Great Britain, *An Act for Preserving the Health of Prisoners in Gaol, and Preventing the Gaol Distemper*, London, 1774.

Green, T. H., and T. H. Grose (eds), [Hume's] *Essays Moral, Political, and Literary*, 2 vols, Darmstadt, 1964.

Greenbaum, Louis S., 'Health-Care and Hospital-Building in Eighteenth-Century France: Reform Proposals of Du Pont de Nemours and Condorcet', *Studies on Voltaire and the Eighteenth Century*, CLII (1976), 895–930.

____'Tempest in the Academy: Jean-Baptiste Le Roy, the Paris Academy of Sciences and the Project of a New Hôtel Dieu', *Archives internationales d'histoire des sciences*, XXIV (1974), 122–40.

Greenberg, Bernard, 'Flies and Disease', *Scientific American*, CCXIII (July 1965), 92–9.

Greenwood, Major, *Medical Statistics from Graunt to Farr*, Cambridge, 1948.

——'Miasma and Contagion', in E. A. Underwood (ed.), *Science, Medicine and History*, London, 1953.

——'Sydenham as an Epidemiologist', *Proceedings of the Royal Society of Medicine: Section of Epidemiology and State Medicine*, XII (1918–19), 55–76.

Guillemeau, J[ean] L[ouis] M[arie], *Coup-d'oeil historique, topographique et médical, sur la ville de Niort et ses environs*, Niort, 1795.

Guillerme, Jacques, 'Le malsain et l'économie de la nature', DHS, IX (1977), 61–72.

Guyton [de] Morveau, L. B., *Traité des moyens de désinfecter l'air, de prévenir la contagion et d'en arrêter les progrès*, Paris, an IX (1800–1).

Hackett, L. W., 'The Disappearance of Malaria in Europe and the United States', *Rivista di parassitologia*, XIII (January 1952), 43–56.

Hacking, Ian, *The Emergence of Probability: A Philosophical Study of Early Ideas about Probability, Induction and Statistical Inference*, London, 1975.

Haeser, H[einrich], *Historisch-pathologische Untersuchungen*, 2 vols, Dresden, 1839–41.

——*Lehrbuch der Geschichte der Medicin und der epidemischen Krankheiten*, 3rd edn, 3 vols, Jena, 1882.

Haguenot, Henri, 'Sur le danger des inhumations', in idem (ed.), *Mélanges curieux et intéressans*, Avignon, 1769.

Hales, Stephen, 'A Further Account of the Success of Ventilators', *The Gentleman's Magazine*, XXIV (1754), 115–16.

——*Statical Essays: Containing Vegetable Staticks; or, an Account of Some Statical Experiments on the Sap in Vegetables*, 2 vols, London, 1731.

——*A Treatise on Ventilators Wherein an Account is Given of the Happy Effects of the Several Trials*, London, 1758.

Hallé, [Jean-Noël], parts of the essay 'Air', in the *Encyclopédie méthodique: médecine*, I, 1787, 492–569; and 'Hygiène', in ibid., VII, 1798, 373–437.

Halley, Edmund, 'A Discourse of the Rule of the Decrease of the Height of the Mercury in the Barometer', PT, no. 179 (January–February 1686), 104–16.

Hannaway, Caroline C., 'The Société Royale de Médecine and Epidemics in the Ancien Régime', BHM, XLVI (May–June 1972), 257–73.

Hannaway, Owen, and Caroline Hannaway, 'La fermature du Cimetière des Innocents', DHS, IX (1977), 181–92.

Hardy, Anne, 'Water and the Search for Public Health in London in the Eighteenth and Nineteenth Centuries', MH, XXVIII (July 1984), 250–82.

Harris, L. E., 'Land Drainage and Reclamation', in Charles Singer *et al.*, (eds), *A History of Technology*, 5 vols, Oxford, 1954–8.

Haviland, Alfred, *Climate, Weather, and Disease*, London, 1855.

Hawkins, F. Bisset, *Elements of Medical Statistics*, Westmead, Farnborough, 1973 reprint, first published 1829.

Haygarth, [John], 'Observations on the Bill of Mortality, in Chester, for the Year 1772', PT, LXIV (1774), 67–78.

_____'Observations on the Population and Diseases of Chester, in the Year 1774', PT, LXVIII (1778), pt I, 131–54.

Heberdeen, William (the elder), 'The Influence of Cold upon the Health of the Inhabitants of London', PT, LXXXVI (1796), pt II, 279–84.

Heberden, William (the younger), *Observations on the Increase and Decrease of Different Diseases*, London, 1801.

Hellmann, Gustav, *Beiträge zur Geschichte der Meteorologie*, 3 vols, Berlin, 1914–22.

Helmuth, J. Henry C., *A Short Account of the Yellow Fever in Philadelphia*, trans. Charles Erdman, Philadelphia, 1794.

Henschen, Folke, *The History and Geography of Diseases*, trans. Joan Tate, New York, 1966.

Herz, Simon, *Versuch einer medicinischen Ortbeschreibung der Ukermärkischen Hauptstadt Prenzlau*, Berlin, 1790.

Hesse, Mary B., *Models and Analogies in Science*, Notre Dame, Indiana, 1966.

Hillary, William, *Observations on the Changes of the Air and the Concomitant Epidemical Diseases, in the Island of Barbados*, 2nd edn, London, 1766; Philadelphia, 1811.

_____*A Practical Essay on the Small-pox*, 2nd edn, London, 1740.

Hindle, Brooke, *The Pursuit of Science in Revolutionary America, 1735–1789*, Chapel Hill, 1956.

Hirsch, August, *Handbook of Geographical and Historical Pathology*, trans. Charles Creighton, 3 vols, London, 1883–6.

Hoffmann, Friedrich (praeses), *Dissertatio inauguralis medica: De morbis certes regionibis et populis propriis*, Halle, 1705 (with J. B. Hoffstadt as respondent).

_____*A Dissertation on Endemial Diseases; or, those Disorders which Arise from Particular Climates*, trans. R. James, London, 1746.

_____*Observationes barometrico-meteorologicae, & epidemicae Hallenses anni MDCC*, Halle, 1701.

Hofsten, Erland, and Hans Lundström, *Swedish Population History: Main Trends from 1750 to 1970*, Stockholm, 1976.

Holmes, Chris, 'Benjamin Rush and the Yellow Fever', BHM, XL (May–June 1966), 246–63.

Home, Francis, *Medical Facts and Experiments*, London, 1759.

Horsfall, William R., *Mosquitoes: Their Bionomics and Relation to Disease*, New York, 1955.

Houttuyn, M[artinus], *Bedenkingen over de sterflijkheid en het getal des volks*, *te Amsterdam, in vergelijking met andere plaatsen*, Amsterdam, 1783.

Howe, G. Melvyn, *Man, Environment and Disease in Britain: A Medical Geography of Britain through the Ages*, New York, 1972.

Huard, P., 'L'emergence de la médecine sociale au XVIIIe siècle', *Concours médicale*, LXXX (18 October 1958), 4 483–6.

Hudson, Robert P., *Disease and Its Control*, Westport, Conn., 1983.

Hull, Charles Henry (ed.), *The Economic Writings of Sir William Petty*, 2 vols, New York, 1963–4 reprint.

Hunter, John, *Observations on the Diseases of the Army in Jamaica*, 2nd edn, London, 1796.

Huxham, John, *Observations on the Air and Epidemic Diseases from the year MDCCXXVIII to MDCCXXXVII*, trans. John Corham Huxham, 2 vols, London, 1759–67.

Huygens, Christiaan, *Oeuvres complètes*, 22 vols, The Hague, 1888–1950.

Jackson, Robert, *A Treatise on the Fevers of Jamaica*, London, 1791.

Jarcho, Saul, 'Cadwallader Colden as a Student of Infectious Diseases', BHM, XXIX (March–April 1955), 99–115.

——'Yellow Fever, Cholera, and the Beginnings of Medical Cartography', JHM, XXV (April 1970), 131–42.

J[aucourt, Louis de], 'Tuyau aérique', in the *Encyclopédie, ou dictionnaire raisonné des sciences*, XVI, 1765, 767–8.

Jones, Colin, and Michael Sonenscher, 'The Social Functions of the Hospital in Eighteenth-Century France', *French Historical Studies*, XIII (Fall 1983), 172–214.

Jones, E. L., 'Disaster Management and Resource Saving in Europe, 1400–1800', in Antoni Mączak and William N. Parker (eds), *Natural Resources in European History*, Washington, 1978.

——*The European Miracle: Environments, Economies, and Geopolitics in the History of Europe and Asia*, Cambridge, 1981.

——and M. E. Falkus, 'Urban Improvement and the English Economy in the Seventeenth and Eighteenth Centuries', *Research in Economic History*, IV (1979), 193–233.

Jones, G. P., 'Thomas Short, an 18th Century Writer on Population', *Yorkshire Bulletin of Economic and Social Research*, VIII (November 1956), 149–58.

Jones, Michael Owen, 'Climate and Disease: The Traveler Describes America', BHM, XLI (May–June 1967), 254–66.

Jordanova, L. J., 'Earth Science and Environmental Medicine: The Synthesis of the Late Enlightenment', in L. J. Jordanova and Roy S. Porter (eds), *Images of the Earth: Essays in the History of the Environmental Sciences* (n.p., 1979).

Journal encyclopédique, Paris, 1762.

Journal oeconomique, Paris, 1762, 1764.

Jurin, James, 'Invitatio ad Observationes Meteorologicas communi consilio instituendas', PT, no. 379 (September–October 1723), 422–7.

Kaiser, Wolfram, 'Die prophylaktische Medizin im halleschen Lehrstoff des 18. Jahrhunderts', *Zeitschrift für Aerztliche Fortbildung* (Jena), LXIII (1 October 1969), 1 062–6.

Keele, Kenneth D., 'The Sydenham–Boyle Theory of Morbific Particles', MH, XVIII (July 1974), 240–8.

Ker, Patrick, 'A Comparison of the Meteorological Registers and Epidemic Diseases at Edinburgh, Rippon, Plymouth, and Norimberg, from May 1731, to June 1736', *Medical Essays and Observations* (abridged), I (1746), 77–96.

Khrgian, A. Kh., *Meteorology: A Historical Survey*, trans. Ron Hardin, 2nd edn rev. Kh. P. Pogosyan, Jerusalem, 1970.

King, Lester S., 'Evidence and its Evaluation in Eighteenth-Century Medicine', BHM, L (Summer 1976), 174–90.

_____(ed. and trans.), *Fundamenta Medicinae* (by Friedrich Hoffmann), London, 1971a.

_____*The Medical World of the Eighteenth Century*, Huntington, N.Y., 1971b, reprint.

_____'Rationalism in Early Eighteenth Century Medicine', JHM, XVIII (July 1963), 1963a, 257–71.

_____ *The Road to Medical Enlightenment, 1650–1695*, London, 1970.

_____'Some Problems of Causality in Eighteenth Century Medicine', BHM, XXXVII (January–February 1963), 1963b, 15–24.

Klein, Herbert S., and Stanley L. Engerman, 'A Note on Mortality in the French Slave Trade in the Eighteenth Century', in Henry A. Gemery and Jan S. Hogendorp (eds), *The Uncommon Market: Essays in the Economic History of the Atlantic Slave Trade*, New York, 1979.

Koller, Armin Hajman, *The Abbé Du Bos: His Advocacy of the Theory of Climate*, Champaign, Ill., 1937.

Kunitz, Stephen J., 'Speculations on the European Mortality Decline', *Economic History Review*, XXXVI (August 1983), 349–64.

La Berge, Ann Fowler, 'A. J. B. Parent-Duchâtelet: Hygienist of Paris, 1821–1836', *Clio Medica*, XII (1977), 279–301.

[La Maillardière, C. F. L. de], *Le produit et le droit des communes, et les intérêts de l'agriculture, population, arts*, Paris, 1782.

Landriani, Marsilio, *Untersuchungen über die Gesundheit der Luft* (trans.), Bern, 1792.

La Roche, R[ené], *Yellow Fever, Considered in its Historical, Pathological, Etiological, and Therapeutical Relations*, 2 vols, Philadelphia, 1855.

Latham, R. G. (ed. and trans.), *The Works of Thomas Sydenham*, 2 vols, London, 1848–50.

Lebrun, François, *Les hommes et la mort en Anjou aux 17e et 18e siècles*, Paris, 1971.

Le Brun, [L. S. D.], *Traité théorique sur les maladies épidémiques dans lequel on examine s'il est possible de les prévoir*, new edn, Paris, 1778.

Lee, W. Robert, 'The Mechanism of Mortality Change in Germany, 1750–1850', *Medizinhistorisches Journal*, XV (1980), 244–68.

Le Fanu, William R., 'The Lost Half-Century in English Medicine, 1700–1750', BHM, XLVI (July–August 1972), 319–48.

Lépecq de La Clôture, [Louis], *Collection d'observations sur les maladies et constitutions épidémiques*, 2 vols, Paris, 1778.

——*Observations sur les maladies épidémiques*, Paris, 1776.

Le Roy, [Jean-Baptiste], 'Observations on the Construction of Hospitals', TAPS, III (1793), 348–50.

Le Roy Ladurie, Emmanuel, *Times of Feast, Times of Famine: A History of Climate since the Year 1000* (trans.), Garden City, N.Y., 1971.

Lesky, Erna, 'Oesterreichisches Gesundheitswesen im Zeitalter des aufgeklärten Absolutismus', *Archiv für österreichische Geschichte*, CXXII (1959), 1–228.

——(ed.), *A System of Complete Medical Police: Selections from Johann Peter Frank*, trans. E. Vilim, Baltimore, 1976.

[Lewis, Thomas], *Seasonable Considerations on the Indecent and Dangerous Custom of Burying in Churches and Church-Yards*, London, 1721.

Liebel, Helen P., *Enlightened Bureaucracy Versus Enlightened Despotism in Baden, 1750–1792*, Philadelphia, 1965.

Lilienfeld, Abraham M. (ed.), *Times, Places, and Persons: Aspects of the History of Epidemiology*, Baltimore, 1980.

Lind, James, *An Essay on Diseases Incidental to Europeans in Hot Climates*, 3rd edn, London, 1777.

——*An Essay on the Most Effectual Means of Preserving the Health of Seamen*, 3rd edn, London, 1779.

Lindeboom, G. A., 'Boerhaave en de oude Griekse geneeskunde', NTG, CVI (6 January 1962), 28–30.

——*A Classified Bibliography of the History of Dutch Medicine, 1900–1974*, The Hague, 1975.

——*Herman Boerhaave: The Man and His Work*, London, 1968.

Lining, John, *A Description of the American Yellow Fever which Prevailed at Charleston . . . in . . . 1748*, Philadelphia, 1799.

——'Extracts of Two Letters', PT, XLII (1742–3), 491–509.

——'A Letter from Dr. John Lining', PT, XLIII (1744–5), 318–30.

——'A Letter from John Lining', PT, XLVIII (1753), pt I, 284–5.

Litton, Edmund, *Philosophical Conjectures on Aereal Influences, the Probable Origin of Diseases*, 2nd edn, London, 1750.

Livi-Bacci, Massimo, 'The Nutrition–Mortality Link in Times Past: A Comment', JIH, XIV (Autumn 1983), 293–8.

Lloyd, Christopher (ed.), *The Health of Seamen: Selections from the Works of Dr. James Lind, Sir Gilbert Blane and Dr. Thomas Trotter*, London, 1965.

——and Jack L. S. Coulter, *Medicine and the Navy, 1200–1900*, Edinburgh, 1961.

Locke, John, 'A Register of the Weather for the Year 1692, Kept at Oates in Essex', PT, XXIV (1705), 1917–37.

Lonie, Iain M., 'Hippocrates Iatromechanist', MH, XXV (1981), 113–50.

De maandelijkse nederlandsche mercurius, Amsterdam, 1759, 1760, 1763.

MacArthur, William P., 'A Brief Story of English Malaria', BMB, VIII (1951), 76–9.

McGlashan, N. D. (ed.), *Medical Geography: Techniques and Field Studies*, London, 1972.

McKeown, Thomas, 'Fertility, Mortality and Causes of Death: An Examination of Issues Related to the Modern Rise of Population', *Population Studies*, XXXII (November 1978), 535–42.

_____'Food, Infection, and Population', JIH, XIV (Autumn 1983), 227–47.

_____*The Modern Rise of Population*, London, 1976.

_____ and R. G. Brown, 'Medical Evidence Related to English Population Changes in the Eighteenth Century', *Population Studies*, IX (November 1955), 119–41.

McManners, John, *Death and the Enlightenment: Changing Attitudes to Death among Christians and Unbelievers in Eighteenth-century France*, Oxford, 1981.

McNeill, William, *Plagues and Peoples*, Garden City, N.Y., 1976.

Magalhães, João Jacinto de, *Description of a Glass-Apparatus . . . together with the Description of Two New Eudiometers*, 3rd edn, London, 1783.

[Mairan], 'Observations météorologiques et botanico-météorologiques', *Histoire de l'Académie royale des sciences* (1743), 20–9.

Maistov, L. E., *Probability Theory: A Historical Sketch*, Samuel Kotz (trans. and ed.), New York, 1974.

Malouin, [Paul-Jacques], 'Histoire des maladies épidémiques de 1746, observées à Paris, en même temps que les différentes temperatures de l'air', *Mémoires de l'Académie royale des sciences* (1746), 220–54.

Manley, Gordon, 'Temperature Trends in England, 1698–1957', *Archiv für Meteorologie, Geophysik und Bioklimatologie*, IX (1959), 413–33.

_____'The Weather and Diseases: Some Eighteenth-Century Contributions to Observational Meteorology', *Notes and Records of the Royal Society of London*, IX (1952), 300–7.

Mathias, Peter, 'Swords and Ploughshares: The Armed Forces, Medicine and Public Health in the Late Eighteenth Century', in J. M. Winter (ed.), *War and Economic Development*, Cambridge, 1975.

Mattock, J. N., and M. C. Lyons (eds and trans.), *Hippocrates: On Endemic Diseases (Airs, Waters and Places)*, Cambridge, 1969.

Mead, Richard, *A Short Discourse Concerning Pestilential Contagion, and the Methods to be Used to Prevent it*, 6th edn, London, 1720.

Menuret [de Chambaud], J[ean] J[acques], *Essai sur la ville d'Hambourg considérée dans ses rapports avec la santé, ou lettres sur l'histoire medico-topographique de cette ville*, Hamburg, 1797.

——*Essais sur l'histoire medico-topographique de Paris*, Paris, 1786.

Meyer, Jean, 'Une enquête de l'Académie de médecine sur les épidémies (1774–1794)', *Annales: ESC, XXI (July–August 1966)*, 729–49.

——'Introduction', in Jean-Paul Desaive *et al.*, *Médecins, climat et épidémies à la fin du XVIIIe siècle*, Paris, 1972.

Michel du Tennetar, *Avis aux messins, sur leur santé, ou mémoire sur l'état habituel de l'atmosphere à Metz*, Nancy, 1778.

Middleton, W. E. Knowles, *The History of the Barometer*, Baltimore, 1964.

——*Invention of the Meteorological Instruments*, Baltimore, 1969.

Millar, John, *Observations on the Management of the Prevailing Diseases in Great Britain*, London, 1779.

——*Observations on the Prevailing Diseases in Great Britain*, London, 1770.

Miller, Genevieve, '"Airs, Waters, and Places" in History', JHM, XVII (January 1962), 129–40.

[Milligen, George], *A Short Description of the Province of South Carolina with an Account of the Air, Weather, and Diseases at Charles-Town*, London, 1770.

Moheau, [Jean-Baptiste], *Recherches et considérations sur la population de la France*, Paris, 1778.

Moivre, Abraham de, *La dottrina degli azzardi*, trans. Roberto Gaeta and Gregorio Fontana, Milan, 1776.

Moreau de la Sarth, Jac[ques] L[ouis], *Esquisse d'un cours d' hygiène*, Paris, [1800?].

——and J[ean] Burdin, *Essay sur la gangrène humide des hôpitaux*, Paris, an V (1796–7).

Morse, Dale L. and Kenneth Rentmeester, 'Death Caused by Fermenting Manure', *Journal of the American Medical Association*, CCXLV (2 January 1981), 63–4.

Moseley, Benjamin, *A Treatise on Tropical Diseases; on Military Operations; and on the Climate of the West-Indies*, London, 1793.

Mossel, J[acob], *Aanmerkingen over Batavia's gesteldheid*, Bavaria, 1753.

Mourgue, J. A., *Essai de statistique*, Paris, [1800].

Muller, O., 'Problèmes de méthodes: Analyse de séries météorologiques anciennes (1776–1792)', in Jean-Paul Desaive *et al.*, *Médecins, climat et épidémies à la fin du XVIIIe siècle*, Paris, 1972.

Muret, Jean Louis, *Mémoire sur l'état de la population dans les pays de Vaud*, Yverdon, 1766.

Nassy, David de Isaac Cohen, *Observations on the Cause, Nature, and Treatment of the Epidemic Disorder, Prevalent in Philadelphia* (trans), Philadelphia, 1793.

Newman, Peter, *Malaria Eradication and Population Growth: With Special Reference to Ceylon and British Guiana*, Ann Arbor, 1965.

Nicolas, [Pierre François], *Histoire des maladies épidémiques qui ont régné dans la province de Dauphiné, depuis l'année 1775*, Grenoble, 1780.

_____*Mémoires sur les maladies épidémiques qui ont régné dans la province de Dauphiné, depuis l'année 1780*, Grenoble, 1786.

Nugent, Thomas (ed. and trans.), *The Spirit of the Laws* [of Montesquieu], New York, 1949.

Oberholzer, Max, *Eine medizinische Geographie der Schweiz aus dem 18. Jahrhundert*, Zurich, 1966.

Ockerse, W. A., *Het begraven der dooden buiten de kerk en stads poorten*, Utrecht, 1792.

Overton, Mark, 'Agricultural Productivity in Eighteenth-Century England: Some Further Speculations', *Economic History Review*, XXXVII (May 1984), 244–51.

Paulet, [Jean Jacques], *Recherches historiques & physiques sur les maladies épizootiques*, 2 vols, Paris, 1775.

Payne, Harry C., *The Philosophes and the People*, New Haven, 1976.

Pearson, Richard, *A Short Account of the Nature and Properties of Different Kinds of Air, so far as Relates to their Medicinal Use*, Birmingham, 1795.

Percival, Thomas, 'Observations on the State of Population in Manchester, and other Adjacent Places', PT, LXIV (1774), pt I, 54–66; LXV (1775), 322–35.

_____*Philosophical, Medical, and Experimental Essays*, London, 1776a.

_____'A Supplement to a Paper, Entitled, Observations on the Population of Manchester', PT, LXVI (1776), 1776b, pt I, 160–7.

Perrenoud, Alfred, *La population de Genève du seizième au début du dix-neuvième siècle: Etude démographique*, 2 vols, Geneva, 1979.

Perrot, Jean-Claude, *Genèse d'une ville moderne: Caen au XVIIIe siècle*, 2 vols, Paris, 1975.

Peter, Jean-Pierre, 'Les mots et les objets de la maladie: Remarques sur les épidémies et la médecine dans la société française de la fin du XVIIIe siècle', *Revue historique*, CCXLVI (1971), 13–38.

_____'Malades et maladies à fin du XVIIIe siècle', in Jean-Paul Desaive *et al.*, *Médecins, climat et épidémies à la fin du XVIIIe siècle*, Paris, 1972.

Petty, William, *Several Essays in Political Arithmetick*, 4th edn, London, 1755.

Peuchet, Jacques, *Statistique élémentaire de la France*, Paris, 1805.

Pfaff, C. H., *Ueber die strengen Winter vorzüglich des achtzehnten Jahrhunderts*, Kiel, 1809.

Philipsborn, Ernst von; 'Geschichte der medizinischen Bioklimatologie', *Medizinische Monatsschrift*, III (1949), 776–9.

Piattoli, Scipione, *An Essay on the Danger of Interments in Cities* (tran.), New York, 1824.

Pointer, John, *A Rational Account of the Weather*, 2nd edn, London, 1738.

Poitevin, Jacques, *Essai sur le climat de Montpellier*, Montpellier, 1803.

[Porée, Charles Gabriel], *Lettres sur la sépulture dans les eglises*, Brussels, 1744.

Porter, Roy, 'The Terraqueous Globe', in G. S. Rousseau and Roy Porter (eds), *The Ferment of Knowledge: Studies in the Historiography of Eighteenth-Century Science*, Cambridge, 1980.

Powell, J. H., *Bring Out Your Dead: The Great Plague of Yellow Fever in Philadelphia in 1793*, Philadelphia, 1949.

Poynter, F. N. L., 'Sydenham's Influence Abroad', MH, XVII (1973), 223–34.

Price, Richard, 'Farther Proofs of the Insolubrity of Marshy Situations', PT, LXIV (1774), 96–8.

Pringle, John, 'An Account of Several Persons Seized with the Gaol-Fever', PT, XLVIII (1753), pt I, 42–54

——*Observations on the Diseases of the Army*, Philadelphia, 1810.

—— 'Some Experiments on Substances Resisting Putrefaction', PT XLVI (1749–50), 480–8, 525–34, 550–8 (with variations in the title).

Puranen, Britt-Inger, *Tuberkulos: En sjukdoms förekomst och dess orsaker, Sverige 1750–1980*, Umeå, 1984.

Ragon, Michel, *The Space of Death: A Study of Funerary Architecture, Decoration, and Urbanism*, trans. Alan Sheridan, Charlottesville, Va., 1983.

Ramazzini, Bernardino, *Constitutionum epidemicarum mutinensium annorum quinque*, 2nd edn, Padua, 1714.

Ramel, M. F. B., *Consultations de médecine, et mémoire sur l'air de Gemenos*, The Hague, 1785.

Ramsay, David, *A Sketch of the Soil, Climate, Weather, and Diseases of South-Carolina*, Charleston, 1796.

Rather, L. J., 'Pathology at Mid-Century: A Reassessment of Thomas Willis and Thomas Sydenham', in Allen G. Debus (ed.), *Medicine in Seventeenth Century England*, Berkeley, 1974.

——'The "Six Things Non-Natural": A Note on the Origins and Fate of a Doctrine and a Phrase', *Clio Medica*, III (1968), 337–47.

Raulin, Joseph, *Des maladies occasionnées par les promptes et fréquentes variations de l'air*, Paris, 1752.

——*Observations de médecine*, Paris, 1754.

Rawlinson, J., 'Sanitary Engineering: Sanitation', in vol. iv of Charles Singer *et al.* (eds), *A History of Technology*, Oxford, 1954–8.

Razoux, [Jean], *Tables nosologiques & météorologiques très-étendues dressés à l'Hôtel-Dieu de Nîmes depuis le 1er juin 1757 jusques au 1er janv. 1762*, Basle, 1767.

Razzell, Peter, 'Population Change in Eighteenth-Century England: A Reinterpretation', *Economic History Review*, XVIII (1965), 312–32.

——*The Conquest of Smallpox*, Firle, Sussex, 1977.

Reinhard, Marcel, André Armengaud, and Jacques Dupâquier, *Histoire générale de la population mondiale*, 3rd edn, Paris, 1968.

Retz, [Noël], *Météorologie appliquée à la médecine et à l'agriculture*, Paris, 1784a.

_____*Précis d'observations, sur la nature, les causes, le symptômes & le traitement des maladies épidémiques que règnent tous les ans à Rochefort*, Paris, 1784b.

Riley, James C., *International Government Finance and the Amsterdam Capital Market, 1740–1815*, Cambridge, 1980.

_____'The Medicine of the Environment in Eighteenth-Century Germany', *Clio Medica*, XVIII (1983), 167–78.

_____'Mortality on Long-Distance Voyages in the Eighteenth Century', *Journal of Economic History*, XLI (September 1981), 651–6.

_____*Population Thought in the Age of the Demographic Revolution*, Durham, N.C., 1985.

Roche, Daniel, 'Talants, raison et sacrifice: L'image du médecin des lumières d'après les éloges de la Société royale de médecine (1776–1789)', *Annales: ESC*, XXXII (1977), 866–86.

Rodschied, Ernst Karl, *Medizinische und chirurgische Bemerkungen über das Klima, die Lebensweise und Krankheiten der Einwohner der holländischen Kolonie Rio Essequebo*, Frankfurt, 1796.

Roekel, G. van, 'Het verzet tegen buitenbegraafplaatsen', NTG, LXXXIV (2 March 1940), 839–41.

Rogers, Joseph, *An Essay on Epidemic Diseases; and More Particularly on the Endemial Epidemics of the City of Cork*, Dublin, 1734.

Rosen, George, 'Cameralism and the Concept of Medical Police', BHM, XXVII (January–February 1953), 1953a, 21–42.

_____'An Eighteenth Century Plan for a National Health Service', BHM, XVI (December 1944), 429–36.

_____*From Medical Police to Social Medicine: Essays on the History of Health Care*, New York, 1974.

_____ *A History of Public Health*, New York, 1958.

_____'Leonhard Ludwig Finke and the First Medical Geography', in E. Ashworth Underwood (ed.), *Science, Medicine and History: Essays . . . in Honour of Charles Singer*, Oxford, 1953b.

_____'Noah Webster: Historical Epidemiologist', JHM, XX (April 1965), 97–114.

_____(ed. and trans.), 'On the Different Kinds of Geographies, but Chiefly on Medical Topographies, and How to Compose Them', BHM, XX (October 1946), 527–38.

_____ 'Problems in the Application of Statistical Analysis to Questions of Health: 1700–1880', BHM, XXIX (January–February 1955), 27–45.

Rosenberg, Charles E., *The Cholera Years: The United States in 1832, 1849, and 1866*, Chicago, 1962.

Royston, Erica, 'A Note on the History of the Graphical Presentation of Data', in E. S. Pearson and M. G. Kendall (eds), *Studies in the History of Statistics and Probability*, London, 1970.

Rush, Benjamin, *An Account of the Bilious Remitting Yellow Fever, as it Appeared in the City of Philadelphia, in the Year 1793*, Philadelphia, 1794.

——— 'An Enquiry into the Cause of the Increase of Bilious and Intermitting Fevers in Pennsylvania, with Hints for Preventing Them', TAPS, I (1786), 206–12.

———'Facts Intended to Prove the Yellow Fever Not to be Contagious', *The Medical Repository*, VI (1803), 135–50.

———*Medical Inquiries and Observations*, 5 vols, various edns, Philadelphia, 1793–1809.

Russell, Alexander, *The Natural History of Aleppo, and Parts Adjacent*, London, 1756.

Russell, Paul F., 'Insects and the Epidemiology of Malaria', *Annual Review of Entomology*, IV (1959), 415–34.

Rutman, Darrett and Anita Rutman, 'Of Agues and Fevers: Malaria in the Early Chesapeake', *William and Mary Quarterly*, 3rd series, XXXIII (January 1976), 31–60.

Rutty, John, *A Chronological History of the Weather and Seasons, and of the Prevailing Diseases in Dublin . . . during the Space of Forty Years*, London, 1770.

Sammlung von Natur- und Medicin- wie auch hierzu gehörigen Kunst- und Literatur-Geschichten, Breslau, 1717–26.

Sand, René, *The Advance to Social Medicine*, London, 1952.

Sarcone, Michele, *Geschichte der Krankheiten die durch das ganze Jahr 1764 in Neapel sind beobachtet worden*, 3 vols, trans. D. J. Th. Schmid von Bellikon, Zurich, 1770–2.

Sargent, Frederick, *Hippocratic Heritage: A History of Ideas about Weather and Human Health*, New York, 1982.

Sauvages [de la Croix], [François] Boissier de, *Dissertation où l'on recherche comment l'air, suivant ses différentes qualités, agit sur le corps humain*, Bordeaux, 1754.

Schnurrer, Friedrich, *Geographische Nosologie, oder die Lehre von den Veränderungen der Krankheiten in den verschiedenen Gegenden der Erde*, Stuttgard, 1813.

Schroeck, Lucas, 'Historia epidemica Germaniae', *Miscellanea curiosa, sive Ephemeridum medico-physicarum Germanicarum Academiae Caesareo-Leopoldinae* (1696), 137–52.

Schwaiger, Albin, *Versuch einer meteorologischen Beschreibung des hohen Peissenbergs als eine nöthige Beylage zu dessen Prospektskarte*, Munich, [1792?].

Schwencke, Thomas, 'Aanmerkingen over het getal der dooden van 1756, 1757 en 1758 in welke twee laatste jaaren kinder-pokjes gegrasseerd hebben in 's Gravenhage', *Verhandelingen uitgegeeven door de Hollandse Maatschappije der Weetenschappen, te Haarlem*, V (1760), 158–67.

Sheynin, O. B., 'On the Early History of the Law of Large Numbers', in E. S. Pearson and M. G. Kendall (eds), *Studies in the History of Statistics and Probability*, London, 1970.

[Short, Thomas], *A General Chronological History of the Air, Weather,*

Seasons, Meteors, &c. in Sundry Places and Different Times; more Particularly for the Space of 250 Years, London, 1749.

Short, Thomas, *New Observations . . . on City, Town, and Country Bills of Mortality*, London, 1750.

_____*A Comparative History of the Increase and Decrease of Mankind in England and Several Countries Abroad*, London, 1767.

Shorter, Edward, *The Making of the Modern Family*, New York, 1975.

Shryock, Richard Harrison, *The Development of Modern Medicine*, Philadelphia, 1936.

_____'The History of Quantification in Medical Science', *Isis*, LII (June 1961), 215–37.

Sigerist, Henry E., 'Problems of Historical–Geographical Pathology', BHM, I (January 1933), 10–18.

Sigsworth, E. M., 'Gateways to Death? Medicine, Hospitals and Mortality, 1700–1850', in Peter Mathias (ed.), *Science and Society, 1600–1900*, Cambridge, 1972.

Simon, Max, *Etude pratique rétrospective et comparée sur le traitement des épidémies au XVIIIe siècle: Appréciation des travaux et éloge de Lépecq de la Clôture*, Paris, 1854.

Sims, James, *Observations on Epidemical Disorders, with Remarks on Nervous and Malignant Fevers*, 2nd edn, London, 1776.

Singer, Dorothea Waley, 'Sir John Pringle and His Circle–Part II, Public Health', *Annals of Science*, VI (1950), 229–61.

Sloane, Hans, *A Voyage to the Islands of Madera, Barbados, Nieves, S. Christophers and Jamaica*, 2 vols, London, 1707–25.

Smith, Dale C., 'Medical Science, Medical Practice, and the Emerging Concept of Typhus in Mid-eighteenth-century Britain', in W. F. Bynum and V. Nutton (eds), *Theories of Fever from Antiquity to the Enlightenment*, London, 1981.

Smith, Wesley D., *The Hippocratic Tradition*, Ithaca, 1979.

Smyth, James Carmichael, *An Account of the Experiment . . . to Determine the Effect of the Nitrous Acid in Destroying Contagion*, London, 1796.

_____[ed.], *The Works of the Late William Stark, M.d. Consisting of Clinical and Anatomical Observations*, London, 1788.

Snorrason, Egill, 'Early History of Medical Climatology', in Sidney Licht (ed.), *Medical Climatology*, Baltimore, 1964.

Société royale de médecine, *Histoire*, 10 vols, Paris, 1776–89.

Staum, Martin S., *Cabanis: Enlightenment and Medical Philosophy in the French Revolution*, Princeton, 1980.

Süssmilch, Johann Peter, *Die göttliche Ordnung in den Veränderungen des menschlichen Geschlechts*, Berlin, 1741; 2nd edn, 2 vols, Berlin, 1761–2.

Susser, M. W., 'The Evolution of Concepts in Epidemiology', in idem, *Causal Thinking in the Health Sciences*, New York, 1973.

[Swift, Jonathan], *Human Ordure, Botanically Considered: The First Essay of the Kind, Ever Published in the World*, London 1748.

Sydenham, Thomas, *Opera medica*, 2 vols, Geneva, 1769.

Tamason, Charles, A., 'From Mortuary to Cemetery: Funeral Riots and Funeral Demonstrations in Lille, 1779–1870', *Social Science History*, IV (1980), 15–31.

Temkin, Owsei, *Galenism: Rise and Decline of a Medical Philosophy*, Ithaca, 1973.

——'Die Krankheitsauffassung von Hippokrates und Sydenham in ihren "Epidemien"', *Archiv für Geschichte der Medizin*, XX (1928), 327–52.

Thiéry, [François], *Observations de physique et de médecine, faites en différens lieux de l'Espagne*, 2 vols, Paris, 1791.

Thijssen, H. F., *Geschiedkundige beschouwing der ziekten in de Nederlanden, in verband met de gesteldheid des lands en de leefwijze der inwoneren*, Amsterdam, 1824.

[Thiroux d'Arconville, Marie Geneviève Charlotte Darlus], *Essai pour servir à l'histoire de la putréfaction*, Paris, 1766.

Thomas, Keith, *Man and the Natural World: Changing Attitudes in England, 1500–1800*, London, 1983.

Thomas, Robert, *Medical Advice to the Inhabitants of Warm Climates*, London, 1790.

Thouret, [Michel Augustin], *Rapport sur les exhumations du cimetière et de l'Église des Saints Innocents*, Paris, 1789.

[Thouvenel, Pierre], *Traité sur le climat de l'Italie considéré sous ses rapports phisiques, météorologiques et médicinaux*, 4 vols, Verona, 1797–8.

Tilly, Louise A., 'The Food Riot as a Form of Political Conflict in France', JIH, II (Summer 1971), 23–57.

Tissot, S. A. D., *An Essay on Bilious Fevers*, (trans.), London, 1760.

Toaldo, Giuseppe, *Essai météorologique sur la véritable influence des astres, des saisons et changemens de tems*, new edn, trans. Joseph Daquin, Chambéry, 1784.

Tournon [Alexandre], *Moyens de rendre parfaitement propres les rues de Paris*, Paris, 1789.

Tourtelle, Etienne, *The Principles of Health*, 2 vols, trans. G. Williamson, Baltimore, 1819.

Towne, Richard, *A Treatise of the Diseases Most Frequent in the West-Indies*, London, 1776.

Tröhler, Ulrich, 'Quantification in British Medicine and Surgery, 1750–1830, with Special Reference to its Introduction into Therapeutics', Ph.D. dissertation, University of London, 1978.

Tromp, S. W., *Medical Biometeorology: Weather, Climate and the Living Organism*, Amsterdam, 1963.

Turner, Michael, 'Agricultural Productivity in England in the Eighteenth Century: Evidence from Crop Yields', *Economic History Review*, 2nd series, XXXV (November 1982), 489–510.

Underwood, E. Ashworth, 'The History of the Quantitative Approach in Medicine', BMB, VII (1950), 265–74.

Vess, David M., *Medical Revolution in France, 1789–1796*, Gainesville, Florida, 1975.

Vetter, Th., 'Essai sur la littérature hippocratique au dix-huitième siècle', in *La collection hippocratique et son rôle dans l'histoire de la médecine*, Leiden, 1975.

Villar[s], D[ominique], *Observations de médecine, sur une fièvre épidémique qui a régné dans le Champsaur & le Valgaudemar en Dauphiné*, Grenoble, 1781.

[Vitet, Louis and Jacques Henri Désiré Petetin], [*Observations sur les maladies régnantes à Lyon*], [Lyon, 1782–4].

Voigt, Gerhard, *Die medizinischen Topographien in Deutschland bis zum Ende des 18. Jahrhunderts*, Berlin, 1939.

Vooys, A. C. de, 'De opkomst van de medische geografie in Nederland', *Geografisch Tijdschrift*, IV (1951), 1–8.

Walker, A[dam], *A Philosophical Estimate of the Causes, Effects, and Cure, of Unwholesome Air in Large Cities*, [London], 1777.

Waring, Joseph Ioor, *A History of Medicine in South Carolina, 1670–1825*, [Charleston], 1964.

——'Lionel Chalmers, Medical Author', BHM, XXXII (July–August 1958), 349–55.

Wasserberg, Franz August Xaver von, *Von dem Nutzen und der Wiese die Luft rein, und die Stadt und Hauser sauber zu halten, besonders bey Gefahr ansteckender Krankheiten*, Vienna, 1772.

Watermann, Rembert, 'Eudiometrie (1772–1805)', *Technikgeschichte*, XXXV (1968), 292–319.

Weaver, George H., 'Life and Writings of William Douglass, M.D. (1691–1752)', *Bulletin of the Society of Medical History of Chicago*, II (1917–21), 229–59.

Webster, Noah, *A Brief History of Epidemic and Pestilential Disease*, 2 vols, New York, 1970 reprint.

——*Letters on Yellow Fever Addressed to Dr. William Currie*, New York, 1979 reprint.

West, Luther S., *The Housefly: Its Natural History, Medical Importance, and Control*, Ithaca, 1951.

White, Paul Dudley and Alfred V. Boursy (eds and trans.), *Translation of De Subitaneis Mortibus (On Sudden Deaths)* (by Giovanni Maria Lancisi), New York, 1971.

White, William, 'Observations on the Bills of Mortality at York', PT, LXXII (1782), 35–43.

Willcox, Walter F. (ed.), *Natural and Political Observations Made Upon the Bills of Mortality* (by John Graunt), Baltimore, 1939.

Winslow, Charles-Edward Amory, *The Conquest of Epidemic Disease*, Princeton, 1943.

——*The History of American Epidemiology*, St Louis, 1952.

——'Jacme d'Agramont and the First of the Plague Tractates', BHM, XXII (November–December 1948), 747–65.

Wintringham, Clifton, *A Treatise of Endemic Disease Wherein the Different Nature of Airs, Situations, Soils, Waters, Diet, &c. are Mechanically Explain'd*, York, 1718.

——*The Works of the Late Clifton Wintringham*, 2 vols, London, 1752.

Wolff, Christian, *Grond-beginzelen van alle de mathematische weetenschappen*, 2 vols, trans. Joan Christoffel van Sprögel, Amsterdam, 1738.

Wolff, Robert Paul (ed.), *The Essential David Hume*, New York; 1969.

Woodward, John, *To Do the Sick No Harm: A Study of the British Voluntary Hospital System to 1875*, London 1974.

Woodward, Theodore E., 'Yellow Fever: From Colonial Philadelphia and Baltimore to the Mid-Twentieth Century', in Abraham M. Lilienfeld (ed.), *Times, Places, and Persons: Aspects of the History of Epidemiology*, Baltimore, 1980.

Wright, Thomas, 'On the Mode Most Easily and Effectually Practicable of Drying up the Marshes of the Maritime Parts of North America', TAPS, IV (1799), 243–6.

Wright, Wilmer Cave (ed. and trans.), *Diseases of Workers* (by Bernardino Ramazzini), New York, 1964.

Wrigley, E. A., and R. S. Schofield, *The Population History of England, 1541–1871*, Cambridge, Mass., 1981.

Index